PRIVATE RENOVATIONS

The facts on
penis
enlargement
options

Dr Ingrid Tall

First published 2022 by Dr Ingrid Tall

Produced by Indie Experts P/L, Australasia
indieexperts.com.au

Cover design by Daniela Catucci @ Catucci Designs
Edited by Anne-Marie Tripp @ Indie Experts
Internal design by Post Pre-press Group, Brisbane
Typeset in 12.5/17 pt Adobe Garamond Pro by Post Pre-press Group, Brisbane
Cover image: from iStock by Getty Images, ID:544797212

ISBN 978-0-6453825-0-1 (paperback)
ISBN 978-0-6453825-1-8 (epub)

Table of Contents

Introduction

We have seen many booms in cosmetic surgery and medicine over the years, and Australians have proven to be firm fans, spending over $1 billion each year on cosmetic procedures – 40% more per capita than the US.[1] It seems almost like no big deal these days for people to have a nip, tuck or lift here and there. If it makes them more confident or more satisfied with their appearance, that's all that counts. The needle has fast replaced the scalpel as the cosmetic surgery tool of choice, though. Dermal fillers and muscle-relaxant anti-wrinkle treatments are the most popular choice in Australia, and it's been estimated that up to 1 in 6 Australian women have had these treatments.[2]

As a general practitioner and cosmetic doctor, I have been injecting filler everywhere on clients' bodies for nearly a quarter of a century. I've injected filler not just into cheeks and lips, but also into necks to lift sagging skin, into ears to rejuvenate earlobes, into scars to smooth them, and into breasts to enlarge them. I have reshaped noses, plumped out gaunt and hollow upper eyelids, treated ageing hands, boosted buttocks, and soothed painful feet with 'stiletto heel' filler. So it's no wonder that filler has also begun to make its way into men's penises.

Penises are simply the next frontier for filler treatments. Even though penis filler is a relatively new treatment, it is certainly the safest and most effective procedure to enhance size – especially compared to some of the often-horrifying techniques that have been tried in the past! I have been performing penis filler treatments for more than five years, and it is one of my favourite procedures due to the positive impact it has on men's lives.

Many men worry about their penis size. They're self-conscious, worrying about what's normal, if they fit in with their peers, if they can please their lovers. Some men find these worries so debilitating that they can't use a public urinal, or are unable to enjoy sexual encounters. Penises come in all shapes and sizes – there are as many small, large, curved, grow-ers, show-ers, colours, fat ones and skinny ones as there are people. When it comes to penis dimensions, size can be a genetic Russian roulette. (By the way, penis size is determined by genes on both the X and Y chromosome, so both of your parents are responsible – you can't blame your mother for everything!) Men have tried all kinds of dangerous or painful things in the quest for a bigger penis, often with devastating results.

With advancements in safe, reversible, long-lasting dermal fillers, however, more and more men are choosing to safely enhance what biology has given them. Even though dermal fillers have been approved for use since the early 2000s, many people are still unaware that *penis* filler even exists. However, I've noticed a growing interest recently, and have been treating more and more clients at my clinic, especially since the start of the COVID-19 pandemic. Recently we had three gentlemen in one day having penis filler. One said, 'If I can't travel overseas during COVID, what else am I going to spend my money on?' It has been quite common for clients to explain that they're undertaking these cosmetic procedures with money saved during the pandemic that they would have otherwise spent elsewhere, or to give themselves a much-needed boost because of the stress caused by the pandemic. I was tempted to call this book *COVID Penis*, but that sounds like a passing fad – all signs point to penis filler being a trend that will persist and grow long after the pandemic is over.

It is pretty nerve-wracking writing a book on penises. I'm sure it will raise eyebrows, and maybe even anger in some people. No-one should be ashamed of their natural body, but no-one should be ashamed if they want to enhance their natural body, either. It can take courage to seek cosmetic treatments, and it takes an extra dose of courage to think about enhancing such a crucially important part of the body like the penis.

Perhaps you picked up this book for a laugh, or because you're curious or even a little bit shocked. Perhaps you're a cosmetic injector wondering about the next big trend. Perhaps you want your partner to have a bigger penis; perhaps you're interested in having some penis filler for yourself. No matter the reason, you will likely have a lot of questions. There are a few I get quite frequently: what type of man actually gets this done? Why do they get it done? What else have men tried in the quest for bigger penises? What is the obsession with penis size, anyway?

I wanted to write this book to explain what penis filler is and how it all works, as well as bust some myths about penis size and enlargements. Read on: this book might just change your life.

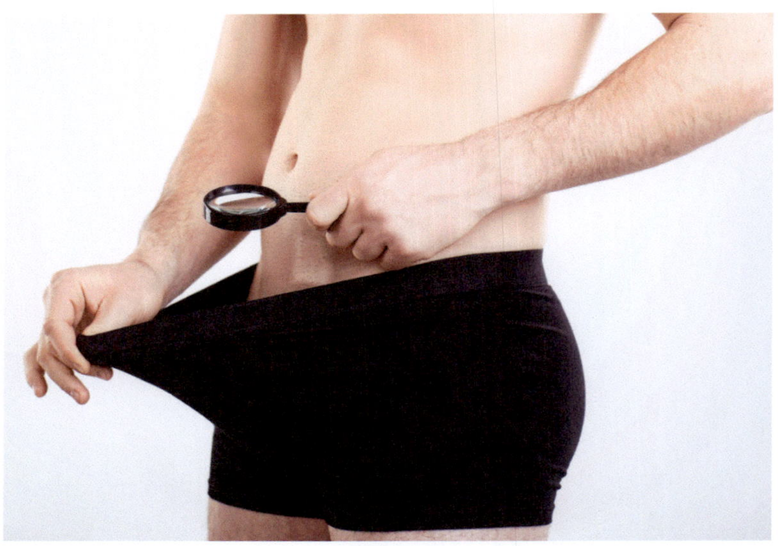

(Studio Romantic/Shutterstock.com)

What's All the Fuss About Penises?

The world marvels that the Eskimos have over fifty different words to describe snow,[3] but there are more than a thousand words for 'penis' in English.[4] The sheer range of vocabulary for genitals – a range that is unparalleled elsewhere in English – which draws upon '[e]very imaginable aspect of the appearance, location, functions, and effects'[5] suggests the degree of power that this singular body part has in our culture, our psyches, and our imaginations.

There has been a historical obsession with penises through the ages – in art, literature, rituals, religion, mythology, fashion and architecture – evident from even the earliest of prehistoric times. Loretta Cormier and Sharyn Jones, in their book *The Domesticated Penis: How Womanhood Has Shaped Manhood*, suggest that the 'importance ascribed to the penis across cultures is so fundamental, frequent, and pervasive that to document all cultural references to the penis would be tantamount to documenting all references to all known human cultures, past and present.'[6] It is useful, though, to note some of the highlights of this history.

Worship

There are depictions of penises in art surviving from the Upper Palaeolithic period (between 40,000–12,000 BCE) in Western Europe. Some of these images appear to depict medical disorders such as phimosis or scrotal masses, while others suggest that foreskin retraction – or even circumcision – was performed.[7] Other images suggest that male genital ornamentation such as tattooing, piercing and scarification were practiced during Paleolithic times, most likely for reasons beyond cosmetic decoration – to show that men were part of a particular community, as part of coming-of-age or other transformative ceremonies, or for spiritual protection or healing.[8]

The ancient Egyptians worshipped a number of phallic gods, including Atum, the original god of Egypt, whose first act was to masturbate to completion, and from his sperm he created all other gods.[9] Called the 'father of the king of Egypt', he was considered the ultimate source of the pharaohs' power as their first ancestor,[10] a clear link between the power of the penis and power in general. Min, the god and 'supreme symbol'[11] of fertility – specifically male fertility – and procreativity, is easily recognisable in Egyptian art: he is usually depicted with a massive erection projecting out from his body.

Penis worship was a big part of ancient Greek and Roman culture, as well. Hermes (Mercury), Pan, Dionysus (Bacchus), and Priapus were all phallic gods, and all also associated with fertility, sexuality, and agriculture in some way. Priapus, perhaps less well known than the others, is quite visually striking – he's depicted as having an oversized, permanent erection. Priapus's image can be found on Roman sculptures, coins, and devotional objects, which were used to invoke fertility and virility.[12] His power as a god of male genitalia is observable in rural Italy even today, with small protective amulets associated with Priapus still used to guard against phimosis.[13]

Erotic, sexual, and phallic imagery abounded in ancient Rome, the extent of which can be imagined from the preserved buildings in the city of Pompeii. Penile imagery was plentiful in Pompeii, including one relief casually displayed outside the local bakery. Phallic statues were erected at Roman city gates for protection and in gardens to encourage the fertile growth of plants. *Facinus*, protective charms or amulets often shaped like an erect penis, were popular with Romans. Images of penises often appeared on jewellery like pendants and rings, household items like lamps or windchimes, or in carvings, and were thought to ward off evil, partly because 'the emotion, shame or laughter, created by obscenity' would divert the threat.[14]

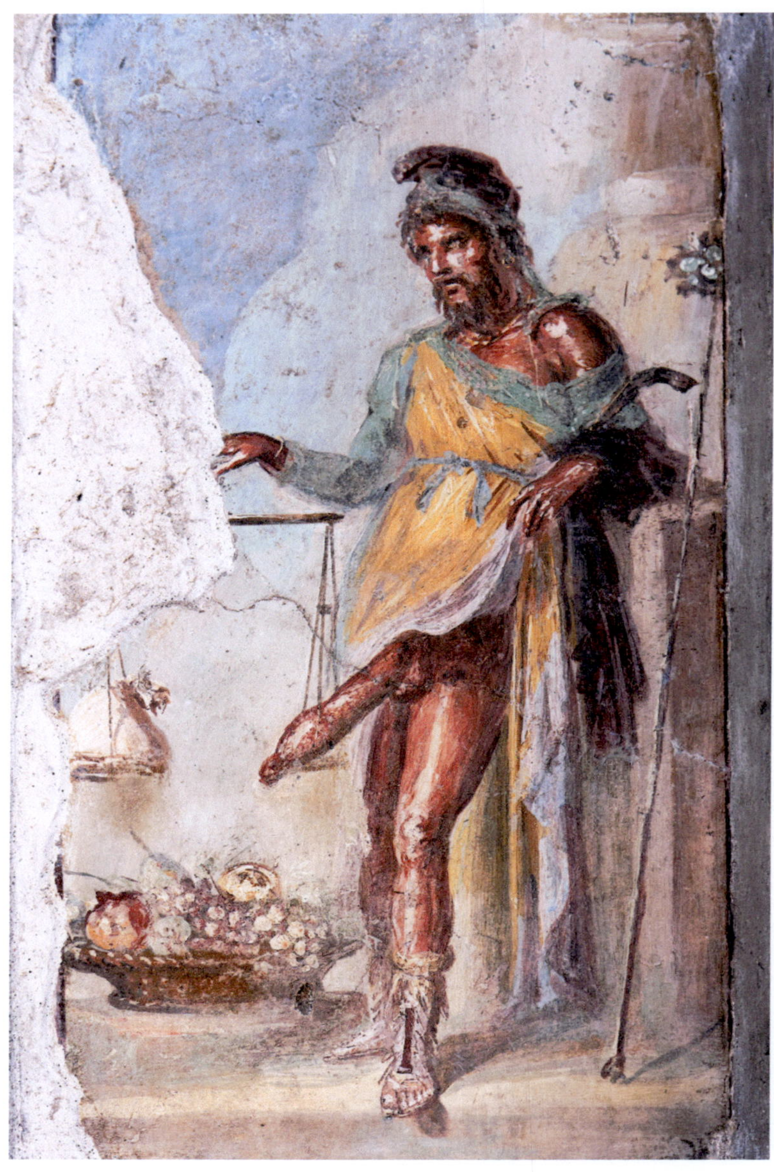

This fresco of the god Priapus, weighing his oversized penis against a bag of money, adorned the foyer wall of the House of the Vettii in Pompeii, Italy. The image is believed to have symbolised the prosperity and status of (or wanted by) the household. (BlackMac/Shutterstock.com)

But have you ever wandered through an art gallery and giggled over the small, flaccid penises sported by ancient statues of heroes and gods? For the Greeks, bigger usually didn't mean better. Big, erect penises were often seen as vulgar and animalistic, associated with drunkenness, a lack of self-control, low intelligence, old age, or foreign 'barbarians'.[15]

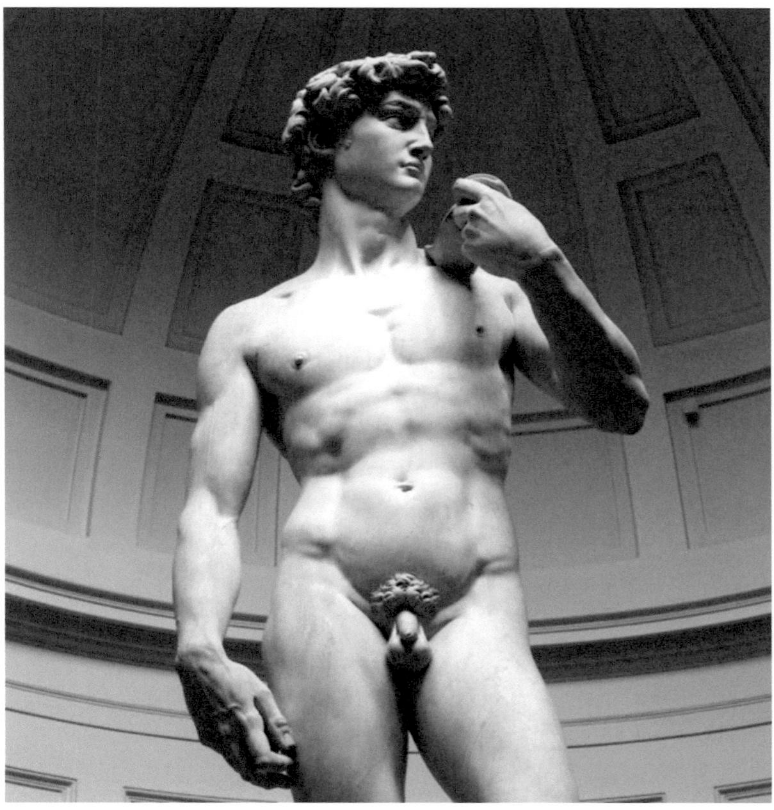

Sculpted in the Renaissance era, Michelangelo's *David* reflected classical Greek ideas of youth, beauty, and strength – including a small penis. (Marta Pons Moreta/Shutterstock.com)

Phallic gods and symbols are or have been worshipped in other world cultures as well – from Kokopelli, a fertility god worshipped by some Native American communities; Chaquen, celebrated as the god of sports and fertility by the Musica civilisation in the Colombian Andes; to Shiva, one of the most important Hindu gods, often represented by a *lingam*, a simple, phallic-shaped object, often embedded in a *yoni*, a lipped, disk-shaped object which may represent the goddess Shakti and female reproductive power.[16] Seasonal festivals in Japan have often incorporated phallic or sexual imagery to invoke or celebrate fertility, sexuality, and good agricultural harvests.[17] One of the most famous of these, which has been celebrated for over fifteen hundred years, is the Hōnen Matsuri (the Harvest Festival), the main procession of which involves moving a 300 kilogram, 2.5 metre-long wooden penis, which is carved new from cypress wood each year, from one shrine to another.[18]

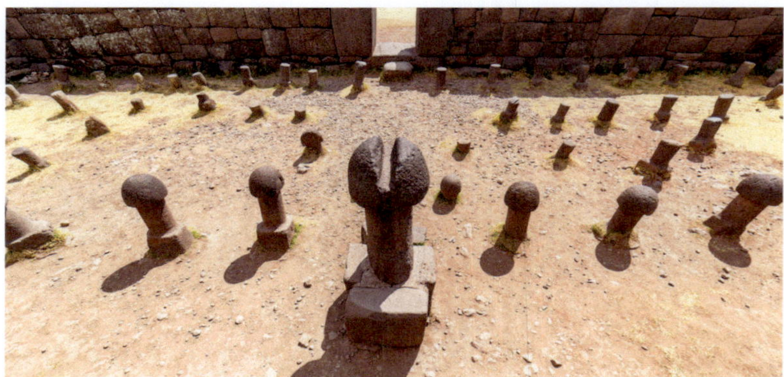

The yard of the Inca Uyo, an ancient temple in Chucuito, Peru, is full of rows of penis-shaped stones, some over a metre high. Local legend has it that this was a site for fertility rituals. (Nicola Messana Photos/Shutterstock.com)

It's understandable why the penis has long been a symbol of fertility, sexuality, regeneration, and creation given its practical role in human procreation. However, some academics argue that the symbolic power of the penis that still influences people today really began around ten thousand years ago, when humans moved away from cooperative hunter-gatherer-style societies to settled, agricultural ones – ones with hierarchical, patriarchal social structures.[19] With agriculturalism came ideas of private property and ownership over land and resources, and ultimately other people – including women. It was at this time that the penis, as the most obvious physical feature separating men and women, began to also symbolise and represent 'male superiority, dominance, and authority'.[20] It's easy to see how the idea that bigger is better may settle into men's minds.

Architecture

Phallic structures and buildings have also been a significant part of penis worship throughout history. For instance, Egyptian obelisks were symbols of creation, with the pillar representing the penis, as well as rebirth, with the pyramidal shape at the top representing a drop of the god Atum's sperm.[21] Tall, vertical structures and buildings are often seen as symbolic representations of the human penis – whether intended to be, or not. Skyscrapers and high-rises, in particular, have been accused of 'dick swinging'. French sociologist Henri Lefebvre argued that the 'arrogant verticality of skyscrapers ... introduces a phallic or more precisely a phallocratic element into the visual realm; the purpose of this display, of this need to impress, is to convey an impression of authority'.[22] Similarly, feminist theorists have commented that high-rise buildings are embodiments of male power fantasies, 'phallic symbols of male domination, power and rational instrumentality.'[23]

The Empire State Building, the Washington Monument, and the Torre Agbar building in Barcelona – among many others – stand tall, dominating their surroundings, bringing to mind the idea of power and authority, but also the image of an erect penis. The tallest building in Brisbane for a few years (2016–2019) housed the executive branch of the Queensland Government; located at 1 William Street, Brisbane, its nickname 'One Big Willy' is a not-so-subtle pun on its address and its penetrative shape.

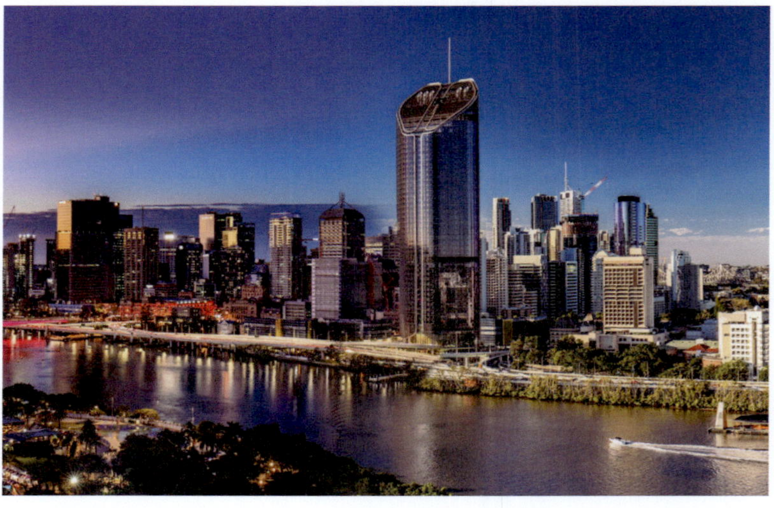

'One Big Willy', one of the tallest buildings in Brisbane's CBD, dominates the skyline. (Martin Valigursky/Shutterstock.com)

Fashion

Fashion trends across cultures and history have also accentuated the importance of the penis. In most cultures around the world, even those which don't require people to clothe themselves fully for modesty or for protection from the elements, the penis is usually covered or sheathed in some way. Penis sheathing is a widely varying cultural practice that, paradoxically, conceals the penis while simultaneously drawing attention to it.[24] The penis sheath was a standout fashion piece in ancient Egyptian; a rectangular flap of fabric worn over the genital area to protect the perceived vital and sacred organ from the elements, including physical injury and diseases.[25] Similar coverings have been depicted in the art of Bronze Age Minoans. Indigenous communities in New Guinea, Vanuatu, the Amazon, and parts of Africa, particularly West Africa, have historically practiced penis sheathing, using gourds, shells, or plant materials as a cover for their genitals.[26]

The men of Pentecost Island, Vanuatu, wear only penis sheaths called 'nanba' when they perform the hair-raising ritual of land diving. I think of these men every time I apply bandages after a penis filler procedure. The ritual is associated with a bountiful yam harvest, and is also a rite of passage for men. The men perform death-defying leaps headfirst from high, hand-built towers with vines tied to their ankles, wearing only their penis sheath strapped tightly to their abdomen. They plunge head-first towards the ground, saved only by the vines around their ankles.

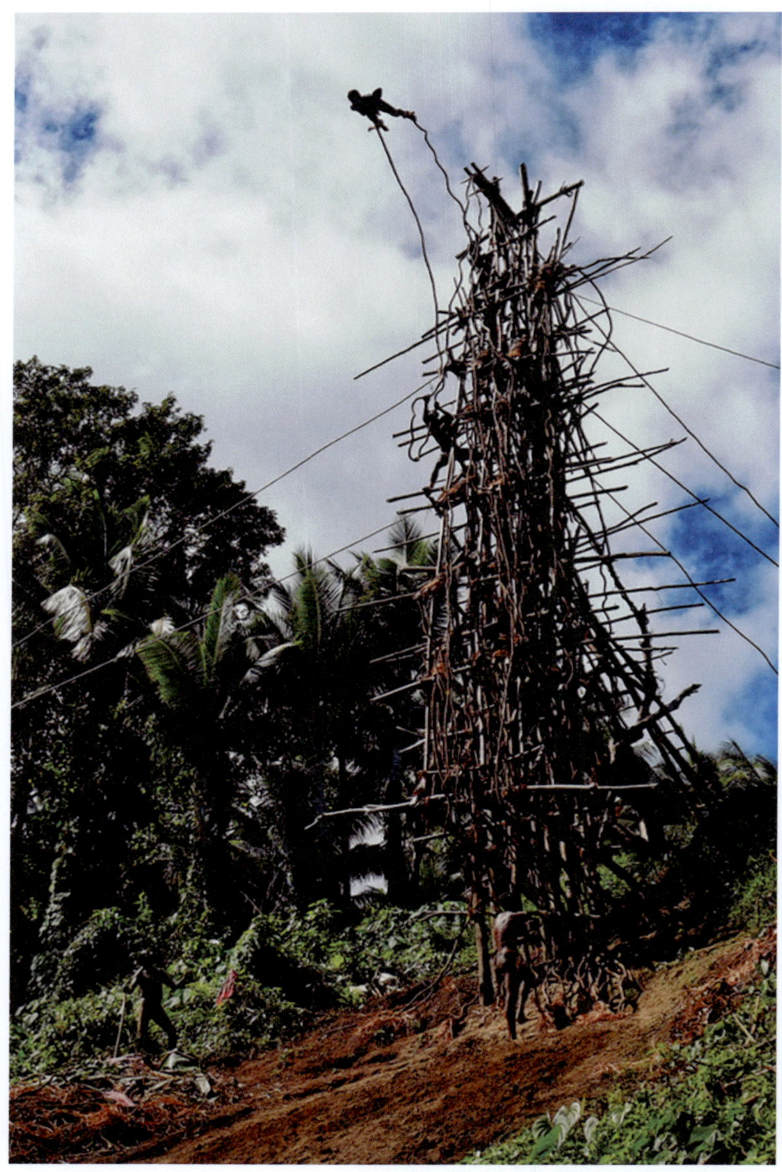

A land diving ceremony on Pentecost Island, Vanuatu, where men leap headfirst from high, hand-built towers wearing only a penis sheath strapped tightly to their abdomen. (Laszlo Mates/Shutterstock.com)

The European codpiece, popular during the European Renaissance, might be considered a type of penis sheath, both covering and accentuating the penis.[27] Between the fourteenth and the sixteenth century in Europe, the simple flap or pouch of fabric attached to the open top of a man's pants to cover his genitals turned into the highly fashionable, heavily padded, elaborately decorated, protruding and exaggerated codpiece, which gave men the appearance of having an 'unnaturally large, semierect' penis.[28] Various theories have been put forward for why codpieces were developed, and why they became so big – they may have been imitations of a piece of military armour, or a way to conceal the messy treatment of syphilis. It may have been a symbol of male power and status – the bigger, more expensively decorated, and less practical codpiece being a way to communicate wealth, occupation, and masculinity. By the end of the sixteenth century, codpieces had fallen out of favour, possibly because of Queen Elizabeth's disdain for them, or because of the influence of King Henry III of France over popular fashions at the time.[29]

While this all seems like ancient history, contemporary men aren't averse to penis-accentuating fashions. Penis 'packing' is a way to make the male organ look more prominent by adding padding – like a sock or two – or a phallic-shaped object into underwear. Some underwear even comes pre-made with strategic padding or support in all the right places, not unlike women's padded or push-up bras.

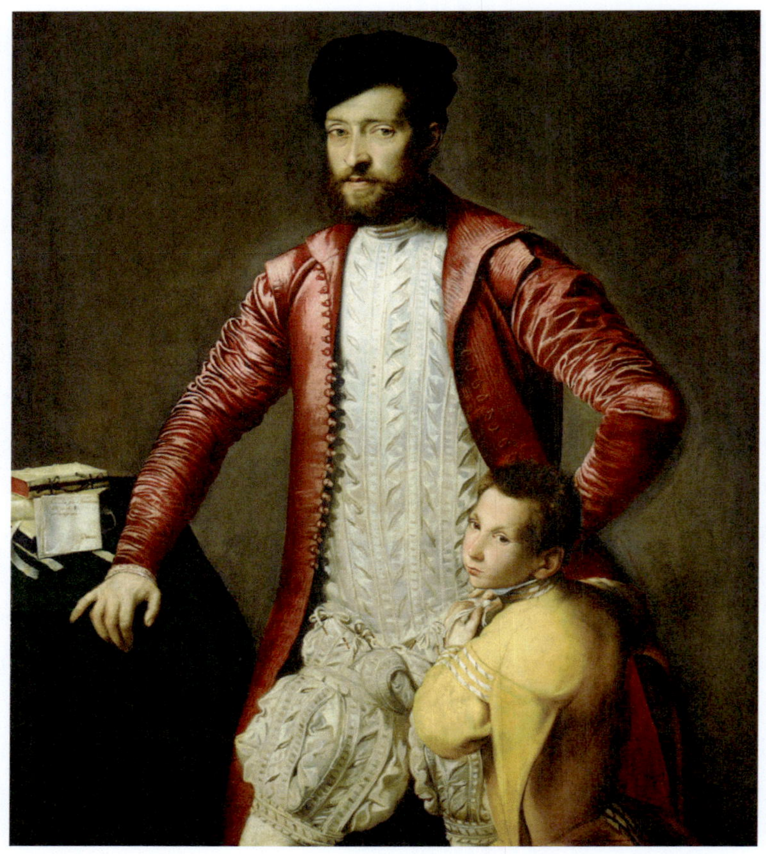

This sixteenth century portrait, attributed to the painter Gian Paolo Pace, shows Florentine nobleman Alessandro Alberti in a fine outfit with a prominent decorative codpiece. Alberti's young page is helping him dress. (Courtesy of the National Gallery of Art, Washington)

Grey sweatpants have also become an unlikely but popular penis-focused fashion item in the past few years. The perfectly mundane, relaxed, casual sweatpants have become a highly sexualised item, thanks to the visible outline of the wearer's penis or bulge that they provide. Between 2015 and 2020, over 1.5 million tweets were made about 'grey sweatpants season'.[30] The norm in many cultures, but especially in the contemporary West, is for the adult penis to be concealed in public, 'particularly from women',[31] which may add to the unexpected eroticism of grey sweatpants – a modest, casual, frequently low-priced fashion item, they conceal the penis completely while also emphasising its presence.

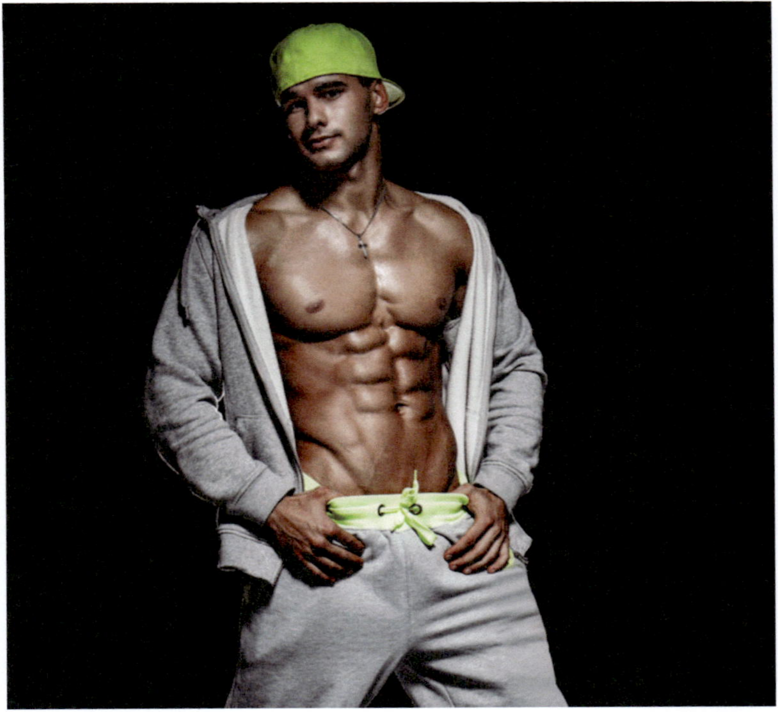

Grey sweatpants – a contemporary penis-focused fashion item. (PawelSierakowski/Shutterstock.com)

Crotch Watching

Perhaps it's no surprise, given the cultural, world-wide obsession with penises, that men and women alike look –

surreptitiously or otherwise – at other men's crotches. *Cosmopolitan* magazine is fairly unashamed about supporting this common habit, featuring articles like 'Celebrity Bulges We Love' and 'The 13 Best Superhero Bulges of All Time',[32] but there's little qualitative research about how widespread this activity is. In a poll by Cosmetic Image Clinics, 66% of respondents confessed to crotch watching – but this figure may have been higher if the survey had been anonymous. Women and men both admitted to casting quick glances at a man's crotch; one woman even swore that she could identify whether a man was circumcised or not. The nurse who conducted the poll, Chris Pokarier, joked that the 34% who said they don't look at men's crotches were 'either religious or lying'.

The risqué images that abound on social media mean that, rather than checking out crotches in real life (and perhaps getting caught looking), people can get their fill in private. Celebrities seem to be capitalising on this habit, at least. A photo golf legend Greg Norman posted of himself and his dog on Instagram went viral in late 2020, because of Norman's wet and clinging boardshorts, and the apparently admiring look on his dog's face at the contents of those shorts. The comments posted on the photo made it clear where people were looking, with fans noting he seemed to be an all-round winner, 'an iron in his hand as well as elsewhere'![33]

Size and Anatomy

Demographics

It's time to get the tape measure out. Do you know what the average size for a penis is? It might surprise you that, even as of 2020, there is no official scientific consensus for measuring penis size.[34] Methods of measurement vary across published studies, as do examination conditions. Some studies depend on men measuring themselves, leading to unreliable results or men embellishing their reported size – when researchers repeated the measuring themselves, penises shrank by around 2.5 cm![35] There is also the possibility that men who volunteer for penis-size studies are more confident with their size than the true average man, skewing averages upwards.[36]

So even if they aren't entirely accurate, what figures do we have for the average penis? One systematic review found that the reported length of a flaccid penis was 'between 7.6 cm and 13 cm in length and 8.5 cm and 10.5 cm in circumference', with an erect length and girth ranging 'between 12.7 cm and 17.7 cm in length and 11.3 cm and 13 cm in circumference.'[37] A different systematic review – which considered twenty different studies of 15,000 men across a range of ages and races – found similar results, concluding that average penis length was 9.16 cm flaccid and 13.12 cm erect, with an average circumference of 9.31 cm and 11.66 cm, flaccid and erect respectively.[38]

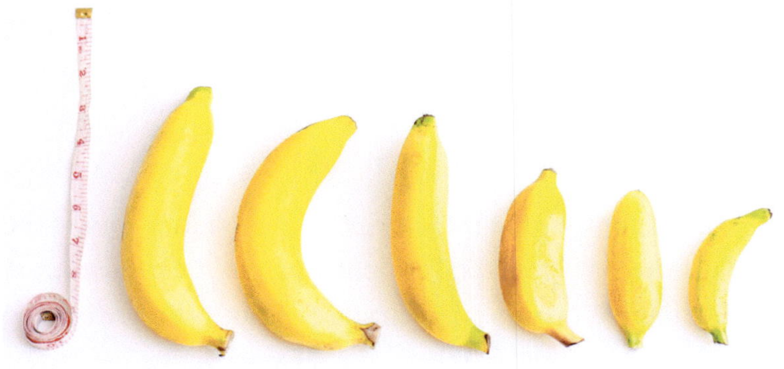

The long and the short of it – do men really know what the average size is? (3623/ Shutterstock.com)

If you're surprised by those numbers, you wouldn't be alone: many men wrongly believe that the average erect penis is greater than 15.24 cm (6 inches).[39] Misunderstandings, misconceptions, and myths around average and desirable penis sizes might explain why so many men feel dissatisfied with their own size. Studies have found that 68.3% of heterosexual adult men and 33.5% of gay and bisexual adult men[40] wished to be bigger; another study of more than 25,000 heterosexual men found that 46% of those who considered their penis to be of average size wished to be larger, with the rate rising to 91% in those who considered themselves small.[41] This study, unfortunately, did not collect demographic questions relating to culture or ethnicity, which the researchers noted may be significant, given 'racial stereotypes about ethnic differences in penis size', and that a person's level of satisfaction with their own size 'may be influenced by his perception of what is typical for his ethnic group.'[42] There are a number of studies that do suggest similar statistics hold true across many parts of the world, though. The Global Online Sexuality Survey, which was launched in 2010 and surveyed Arabic speakers in the Middle East, found that '[d]issatisfaction with length affected 41% of participants, girth affected 15%, and dissatisfaction with both affected 44% of individuals.'[43]

One researcher has suggested that if men were more frequently educated about average penis size (including the flaws in so many studies about size), it could correct their misconceptions about average size, correct any false beliefs they had about their own size, and confirm that they are completely normal – and unlikely to be in any need of medical intervention or enlargement.[44]

What about the outliers? A penis less than 7 cm in the erect state is defined as a micropenis. Only 0.6% of men have a micropenis, and while it is usually a result of genetics, it may also be a result of a hormonal condition. Micropenis might sound like the poor cousin of a comic book superhero, but it might be a case of small but mighty, as micropenises – generally – still work productively. A penis greater than 5 cm is capable of penetrative intercourse and repro-duction – and pleasure.

Small penis syndrome

Worrying about penis size can be a normal experience for men, especially as so few men know the facts and figures around average penis size. However, sometimes this worry becomes pathological and excessive with rumination and generalised anxiety to the point where the condition is medi-calised, with a label of small penis syndrome (SPS) or small penis anxiety (SPA).

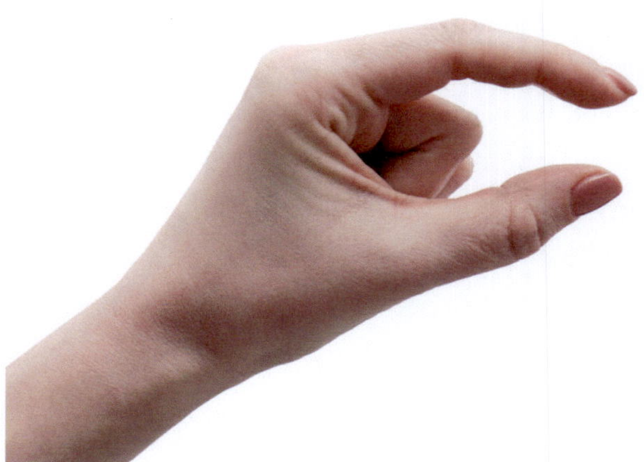

A pathological and excessive fear of having a small penis may be a case of small penis syndrome or small penis anxiety. (Tverdokhlib/Shutterstock.com)

Small penis syndrome is defined as 'anxiety about the genitals being observed, directly or indirectly (when clothed), because of concern that the flaccid penis length and/or its girth is less than the normal for an adult male, despite evidence from a clinical examination to counter this.'[45] Even though men who experience SPS generally have completely normal sized penises, this can be a distressing and debilitating syndrome.[46] A man with SPS might avoid situations where his penis becomes partially or fully visible in order to avoid imagined ridicule – like sexual relationships or encounters; swimming, the gym, communal showers or urinals; even seeking medical diagnosis or treatments. If a man experiences SPS, it can have major flow-on effects with his self-esteem, his sexual well-being, and his sexual and social relationships – it can be difficult wearing your genitalia on the outside.

It is common for boys to have doubts about whether they are large enough in change rooms at school, and similarly with men when they are in a gym, locker room, or while standing at the urinal with other men. It astonishes me how often in American movies there is a scene involving two men holding their penises, standing at a urinal and talking to each other. The 'urinal' location scene can be symbolic of camaraderie and intimacy but often it is more symbolic of one-upmanship or competition, of 'sizing each other up'. One client told me that guys 'always' take a quick, furtive glance to check out the size of other men using urinals, and that he often feels inadequate in this scenario.

Research suggests that approximately two-thirds of men with SPS recall that the problem started in childhood when they thought their penis was smaller than their friends', especially friends who developed secondary sexual characteristics earlier than they did.[47] The remaining one-third report noticing that the problem developed in their teenage years when they started looking at erotic images or pornography. Pornography is more accessible than ever before: what were once racy magazines hidden under the bed to be found by a mother or diligent cleaner is now an incognito browser accessed at the speed of a finger-click. The constant presence of smart phones with internet accessibility in our contemporary lives means that pornography can be accessed all the time, and anywhere. To compare oneself to pornstars, particularly those with larger-than-average penises, may be particularly depressing for men.[48]

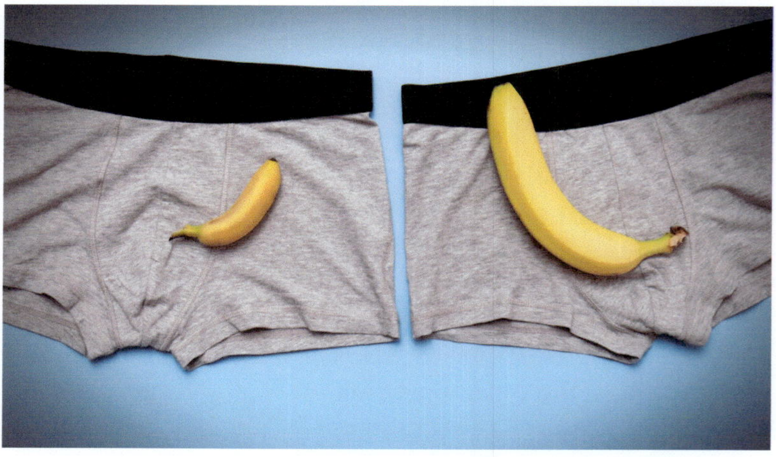

Many men's experience of small penis syndrome begins at a young age, when they begin comparing themselves to their peers. (RealPeopleStudio/Shutterstock.com)

Studies also suggest that men who have received negative comments, particularly from peers or sexual partners, about their penile appearances are more prone to self-dissatisfaction or SPS, and are more likely to consider enhancement procedures such as medications, creams, pumps and surgery.

Small penis syndrome may be a manifestation of body dysmorphic disorder (BDD), which it is estimated to affect about 2.5% of the population. With BDD, a person focuses on imagined or minor flaws and builds them up causing distress and anxiety. Sometimes this BDD focuses on the appearance of the genitals. And let's face it, small penises are often – unfairly – picked on in society. Comments and jokes about small penises abound in TV shows and movies, where men are teased and emasculated about the size of their penis, with the topic offering 'great inspiration for caricaturists and comedians'.[49]

Cognitive behavioural therapy can be productive in building confidence and self-esteem for those suffering from SPS or BDD, but sadly, many men may avoid seeking help.[50]

Big feet and other old wives' tales

I was assisting during a caesarean section one day, and when the baby was pulled out of the mum's belly everyone was startled by the big feet of this newborn baby. The attending obstetrician joked, 'You know what they say about large feet?' Everyone waited with bated breath for the answer. 'Large feet, large shoes,' he said. He was clearly not a believer in the popular folk theory that foot size meant anything about other body parts.

If you have a smaller (or larger) than average penis, would someone be able to tell this from your other physical characteristics? It is often suggested that a person's penis size might correlate with the size of their hands or feet, their overall height, or the size of their nose. One Korean study suggests that men with longer ring fingers compared to their index fingers have slightly longer penises,[51] while another study found a correlation between the 'size of the stretched penis and foot size and height' but concluded that the correlation 'was too weak to be used as a practical estimator.'[52] Another study found no relationship between the size of the foot and penis size, stating 'the supposed association of penile length and shoe size has no scientific basis.'[53]

If you can't tell how big someone's penis is by their shoe size, does having a longer flaccid penis mean you have a bigger erection? The size of the flaccid penis does not predict or correspond to erectile length, which may seem surprising.[54] Some smaller flaccid penises grow much longer, while some larger flaccid penises grow comparatively less. This has led to the saying 'I'm a grower, not a shower.'

When we talk about penis size, it's hard to avoid jokes or insinuations about race and size – that penile size varies from race to race, and specifically that black people have bigger penises.[55] This myth, and the studies which argue for it, are unfortunately based in 'vulgar racial stereotypes' and pseudoscience,[56] but sadly continue to be perpetuated – even in clients I see. Three Afghani men recently presented to my clinic requesting penis filler, while blaming the marauding Asian barbarians who stormed into their country centuries ago for the smallish magnitude of their penises. However, researchers have concluded that while there are 'no indications of differences in racial variability' of penis size in academic studies, it is not currently possible to draw any conclusions about size and race from the available literature and that further research may need to be conducted.[57] Other studies report the same – that no scientific evidence exists to support the idea that penis size varies significantly between races, or the myth that black people in particular have over-sized penises.[58]

What about the idea that penises shrink as we age? If you live long enough, could you end up with a micropenis? Many men believe their penises will shrink or have shrunk with age but again, science seems to fly in the face of populist opinion and personal observations. One client swore that his erection used to extend to his belly button but over the years it had lost a few centimetres. Some individual research studies have suggested that penis size is smaller in older men, but a systematic review of the results of numerous studies over a 60-year period found no overall difference in size linked to ageing.[59] There is no evidence to suggest that penises shrink with age, even though some people do lose a bit of overall height as they get older. The testicles and scrotum, though, do sag as age approaches due to loss of elasticity in the skin. Saggy testicles are natural and this could make the penis look smaller due to the increased relative lengthening of the scrotal sac.

Other syndromes

Another reason why people may think that their penis is shrinking with age is because of middle-aged weight gain and buried penis syndrome. Humans have a fat pad above the pubic bone called the mons pubis, or mons Venus in women, which has a shock-absorbing and cushioning role. As people gain weight, this fat pad increases in size. As it increases for men, it surrounds and envelops the base or root of their penis. As the base of the penile shaft becomes buried in this mound of fat, the penis looks as if it is shorter than it really is, just like a house can look low-set when encased in snow. The more fat in this fat pad, the smaller the penis will appear. If you push down on the fat on top of your pubic bone, you will see a significant amount of the penis shaft revealed. While buried penis syndrome can be acquired later in life thanks to 'middle aged spread', it can occur in boys and men at any age from birth, as a result of excessive skin, fat, or connective tissue, or due to abnormalities in connective fascia and ligaments.[60]

It is nice to know that if you are overweight and you feel your penis falls short of your tape measure aspirations, one of the cheapest and most effective ways to increase your length is to simply lose weight. Other treatments for buried penis syndrome include fat removal using either fat freezing techniques such as Coolsculpting™, radiofrequency heating of fat cells, and fat dissolving injections containing a bile acid similar to the digestive enzymes that breaks down the fat in your gut.

So you might not be too worried about a little extra fat making your penis look a bit shorter – but have you ever worried that your penis would disappear entirely? It sounds like a bizarre joke, but this is a real delusion experienced by some people. Delusions of this type can affect individuals or even whole groups of people when they think their penis is shrinking or disappearing. This is known as shrinking penis syndrome, penis panic or Koro – a Malay word meaning 'head of a turtle', referring to when a turtle retracts their head into their shell. (The word sounds similar to 'Kuru', a viral disease found in Papua New Guinea caused by eating human brains, but rest assured eating human brains does not cause the psychiatric delusional state of 'Honey, I shrunk my penis'!)

Shrinking penis syndrome can be a very distressing condition. Sufferers can experience a fear of impending death, the loss of sexual power, and an overwhelming belief that their penis is actually shrinking and will soon disappear. Outbreaks of mass hysteria relating to Koro have occurred around the world, including in Europe, Africa, Asia, and the United States. In 1967, ninety-seven people in Singapore were hospitalised in a single day after a news report said that some people were developing the condition after eating the meat from pigs that had been vaccinated against swine flu.

Similar delusions existed in the Middle Ages in Europe, where it was believed that witches had the power to emasculate men. The fifteenth century treatise on witchcraft, the *Malleus Maleficarum*, included stories about men who claimed that their genitals had vanished, being 'hidden by the devil … so that they can be neither seen nor felt.' When the witches were placated, the men's genitals reappeared.

Luckily, shrinking penis syndrome is rare, and treatment with either psychotherapy or anatomical education seem to be quite successful.

What Do Women and Men Who Have Sex with Men Want?

Some of the anxiety men feel about their penis size may by driven by their beliefs about what their sexual partners want, and their fears that they may not be sexually satisfying. One of the most frequently given reasons by men seeking penile enhancement procedures is their 'desire to "dazzle" women.'[61] But these fears and beliefs may not be accurate, meaning this anxiety is completely unnecessary. A 2014 study found that while both men and women estimated the ideal size of an erect penis to be larger than the average size, men's estimates of what *they thought* women considered ideal were significantly greater than the estimated ideal actually given by women.[62] So what do women want?

One large study of 52,000 heterosexual men and women found that 85% of women were satisfied with the size of their partner's penis.[63] By comparison, only 55% of men were satisfied with their own size. Only 6% of the women surveyed considered their partner's penis to be small, with most women (67%) rating their partner's penis as average sized. Only 14% of women wished their partner's penis was larger.

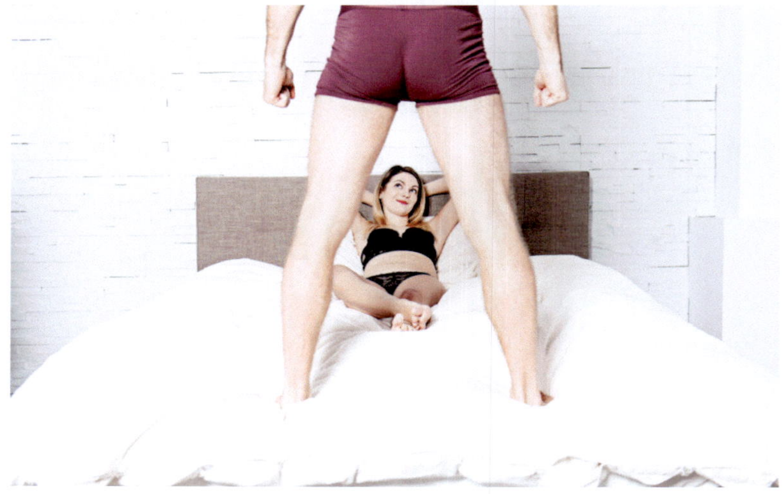

The desire to dazzle a sexual partner can be compelling. (Lopolo/Shutterstock.com)

Another study suggests that, for women in heterosexual relationships, girth is more important than length when it comes to penis size and sexual satisfaction – 33% of women surveyed said girth was important, compared to 21% of women who said the same of length.[64] A more interesting figure to come out of this study might be that 77% of women surveyed said that penis length was unimportant or totally unimportant to their sexual satisfaction, as did 67% of women regarding girth.

However, researchers have also noted that women's preferences may change depending on relationship context, finding that women prefer a penis of slightly larger-than-average circumference and length for a one-time sexual encounter, while preferring average- or smaller-sized penises within a long-term, stable relationship.[65] This is all for good, physiological reason. While the pleasure offered by a larger, girthier penis might be attractive for a single sexual encounter partly because the 'increased physical sensation compensates for the reduced psychological connection',[66] women are more likely to seek out a penis which is less likely to cause them discomfort, pain, or physical damage for regular, long-term sexual partners. The vagina is an incredibly complex organ, comprised of very elastic, stretchy tissue; it can keep a slender tampon in place, but also expand to stretch around a penis during intercourse, or a baby during labour. The vagina is about 6–8 cm deep on average, and increases to 10.8–12 cm when aroused.[67] Stretch receptors proliferate in vaginal tissue and they are stimulated naturally by the penis, and, just as a large meal stimulates the stretch receptors in your stomach making you feel contented, a larger penis may stimulate these stretch receptors more – but this creates pleasure only up to a point, beyond which lies discomfort or pain. Despite this, men often wish for dimensions that won't easily be accommodated by an 'average' vagina[68] – but there is no point being so well endowed that you're not able to use it. For heterosexual sex, a penis being longer than the vagina may be a waste of biological real estate.

While some women who do reach orgasm through penetrative sex may rate penis size as more important than those who don't,[69] the real powerhouse of female sexual pleasure is the clitoris, particularly direct stimulation of the clitoris by the male mons pubis and pubic bone during intercourse, rather than the penis. However, in one study of 303 American women, penetrative intercourse was deemed only a slightly better trigger for orgasm (62%) than external stimulation by their partner's mouth or hand (both 48%).[70]

The broader context of a sexual encounter or sexual relationship may also be more important to sexual pleasure than the size of a single organ, particularly in long-term sexual relationships. One study of sexual satisfaction found that for both men and women in long-term heterosexual relationships, their satisfaction with the non-sexual aspects of their relationship was a much better indicator of their overall sexual satisfaction than their reported satisfaction with their actual sexual interactions.[71]

Unfortunately, there are very few similar studies of what men who have sex with other men consider to be an ideal, desirable penis size in a partner. One survey found that only 7% of gay men considered the penis to be their favourite feature of another man's body, and the men surveyed gave vastly mixed responses about how important (or not) penis size was to them.[72] In an online poll of over 550 gay and bisexual men, more men said that penis size *didn't* matter than those who said it did (49% to 37%).[73] Around a fifth of the men in this poll said that they had turned down sex with someone because of their penis size – but this figure included those who rejected a partner whose penis they considered to be too big, not just too small.

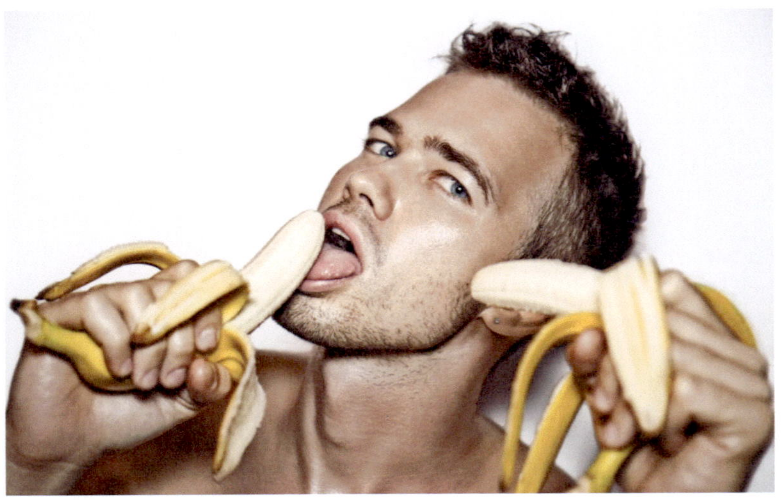

Just one tool in the pursuit of giving and getting pleasure. (Elquest/Shutterstock.com)

Penis size may be more important to some gay men because of the 'erotic nature of the body in many gay cultures and the "double presence" of the penis in a gay relationship or sexual encounter' and the 'overall importance of the body in dominant gay male culture, especially as a site of erotic symbolism.'[74] However, one online column offered this valuable, thought-provoking advice to a young gay man nervous about his size: 'Your penis is just one tool … can you think beyond your penis to all the ways you could possibly give pleasure, get pleasure and connect to another person?'[75]

Penis Enlargement Options – the Good and the Bad

People will go to great extremes to allay anxiety about their penis size. The holy grail of a safe, economical, effective method to make this penis larger – longer, wider, or both – has been elusive but people have been adventurous and spirited in their plight, in past and modern times. Some attempts have been quite simple; some have involved hugely invasive surgeries. Some attempts have simply been a waste of time and money. Some attempts have had devastating physical consequences. But men (and their doctors) have nevertheless been dogged and persistent in their efforts to find this holy grail, and one option – hyaluronic dermal filler – may just be it. Let's take a look at some of the attempts and options that men have tried.

Pills and pumps

The sheer number of 'increase your inches' spam messages that appear in email inboxes are testament to the persistent anxiety around size in many men's minds. All kinds of lotions, potions, pills, supplements, pumps, exercises, and tools are advertised, promising often extreme increases in length, girth, and/or sexual stamina – and it's easy to see why they might be tempting. They're often inexpensive, they're a quick and easy fix, often advertised as 'safe' or 'natural' options, and are able to be used alone in the privacy of your own home. But do any of them actually work? The short answer is no – and in fact they may be counterproductive, or cause damage or injury to your penis.

In Australia, most supplements are not required to pass the same level of testing or regulation as prescription medicines before they are sold. The Therapeutic Goods Administration (TGA), which oversees the regulation of medicines in Australia, relies on manufacturers to simply be honest in reporting the ingredients they use, the quality of those ingredients, and their manufacturing process. The TGA also doesn't require any proof from manufacturers that the products they're selling actually work.[76] This means that you can never be quite sure that your supplement actually contains any of the promised ingredients, whether it contains unlisted or dangerous ingredients, or if it will ever work. But when supplements are sold online, it's likely they haven't been through any TGA evaluation at all. Even if the supplements do contain only the ingredients on the label, there is no evidence to show any link between the common herbal inclusions – like maca, horny goat weed, and ginkgo biloba – and sexual function; but there is evidence that they can cause negative health effects like anxiety, mood swings, and hallucinations.[77]

You might think that supplements containing hormones like testosterone might be more effective. Penis tissue has no bio-active hormone within it; it is the testicles which produce the hormone testosterone, which causes men's genitals to develop during puberty and produce sperm, as well as maintains libido, muscle strength and bone density. The hypothalamus, a gland in the brain which controls hormone production, sends signals to the pituitary gland to secrete hormones which cause the testicles to produce more testosterone. But it's a delicate feedback system. If too much exogenous testosterone (testosterone from external sources) is taken into the body, the hypothalamus alerts the pituitary gland to suppress hormone production, and the testes will stop producing testosterone. The testicles can shrink with the lessened burden of testosterone production in the feedback loop mechanism, becoming like soft, flabby grapes. Not the desired outcome!

External physical tools like vacuum pumps, penile traction extenders and peno-scrotal rings also get touted for their ability to increase size. Vacuum pumps have been around for a long time, first suggested as a solution for erectile dysfunction back in 1874.[78] These pumps use negative pressure to draw blood into the penis, thus expanding it. There is evidence that vacuum pumps do encourage erections and may be a successful treatment for erectile dysfunction, and they may cause a temporary and small boost to penis size because of the extra blood which has been drawn into the area. However, there is no evidence to show that they are effective in permanently enlarging the penis in any way.[79] Using a penis pump incorrectly or too frequently may cause pain, bruising, numbness, burst blood vessels, or permanent damage to the tissue of the penis.[80]

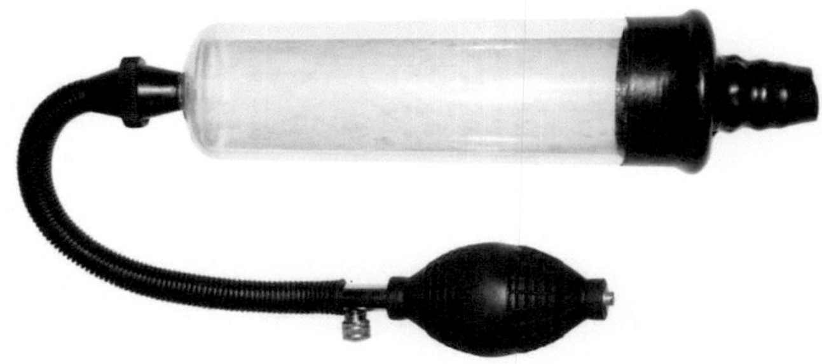

An example of a manual vacuum penis pump, which uses negative pressure to draw blood into the penis. They may give a temporary, small boost to penis size, but can be risky if used incorrectly. (begun1983/Shutterstock.com)

Similarly, peno-scrotal rings may have temporary, short-term benefits in increasing erection size, but there is no scientific evidence to suggest their use causes long-term penile enlargement. Peno-scrotal rings are rings made of rubber, metal or leather which can be strapped around the penis and scrotum during an erection. They are designed to enhance erectile staying power, and like penis pumps may give a temporary and minor boost to penile size due to blood engorgement. However, one of the big risks include 'penile incarceration', or strangulation, which was first reported back in 1755.[81] Penile incarceration can lead to kidney failure, death, or gangrene which might cause the penis to drop off entirely.

DIY penis lengthening exercises like 'milking' or 'jelqing' have also been touted, especially on the internet, for their potential to add length. These are exercises that involve repeatedly pulling on the flaccid or semi-flaccid penis using your hand to encourage the connective tissue in the penis to stretch or relax. However, there is no scientific evidence that these manual 'do it yourself' exercises can be successful in increasing the length or girth of the penis, but there is evidence that they may cause bruising, swelling, numbness or tearing of the delicate blood vessels and veins.[82]

'Slow grow' penile traction extension devices appear to have the most evidence supporting their success. They have been used throughout history, across many cultures.[83] Penile traction extension devices are mechanical contraptions attached to the shaft of the penis, and apply gentle but progressive tension in order to painlessly stretch the penis tissue and increase the length of the penis through soft tissue cellular proliferation. Penis extenders have to be worn every day for some months, and for between four to six hours every day, and if used consistently and correctly, may return good results.[84] One study found that men gained an average of 2.3 cm to the length of their flaccid penis after using one device for at least four hours every day for six months;[85] another study reported an average increase of just under

2 cm to flaccid length after three months, with participants wearing the device for four to six hours for the first two weeks, and then nine hours a day for the remainder of the study.[86] While, unfortunately, no girth increase is achieved by applying traction forces, there has thankfully also been no recorded reduction in girth. Even though these are positive results, they are hard earned, requiring a great deal of commitment over a long period of time.

Surgical options

Surgery has been the backbone of penis enlargement endeavours for medical purposes since the first recorded successful surgical penile augmentation in 1971,[87] but it is only for the very committed – the thought of a scalpel wending its way through the nether regions is a too much for many to bear! Surgical enlargement options for cosmetic purposes are generally considered experimental, highly risky, ineffective, and potentially damaging to a patient's mental and physical health.[88] Even surgeons performing and promoting surgical enlargements comment that it 'very rarely produces spectacular results'.[89] While the Australian Medical Association notes that a range of health conditions may merit genital surgery, they strongly urge against genital surgeries for cosmetic reasons, citing 'a lack of data supporting the benefits … and a range of potential complications and adverse outcomes [which] have been associated with these procedures.' The Mayo Clinic puts it more bluntly: 'no reputable medical organisation endorses penis surgery for purely cosmetic purposes.'[90] The American Urological Association's position is that a micropenis is the only legitimate reason for penis enlargement surgery,[91] but research shows that most men seeking these surgeries have completely normally-sized and normally-functioning penises.[92] Despite the risks and medical warnings, interest in cosmetic penile enlargement surgeries has increased over the past few decades.[93]

Surgical options, also known as augmentation phalloplasty, include techniques such as cutting the suspensory ligament of the penis, fat transfer injections, and dermal-fat skin grafting. The most common surgical procedure for penis lengthening involves cutting the penis' suspensory ligament. This ligament attaches the top of the penis to the pubic bone; it holds the penis up snugly against the pubic bone, and supports and stabilises the penis when it's erect.[94] Cutting this ligament allows the penis to drop away from the pubic bone and hang down further. Cutting the suspensory ligament has no impact on the length of the erect penis, but may result in an increase of 1–3 cm when it's flaccid – but results may be inconsistent and no increase in length is guaranteed.[95] The release of the suspensory ligament often also requires skin reconstruction to accommodate the new extra penile length, which may lead to complications such as disrupted blood supply to the penis and scarring around the pubic area and base of the penis.[96] Patients may also have to hang weights of at least 4.5 kilograms from their penis to encourage lengthening and ensure the ligament does not reattach over a period of months to years after the operation.[97]

Ligaments exist in our bodies for a good reason, so the risks of this surgery are significant. One risk is that the suspensory ligament may heal and reattach to the pubic bone at a higher point, resulting in a shorter penis.[98] It may also lead to the loss of sensation in the penis; a loss of stability, support, and upward angle during erection causing difficulty with penetration and other sexual activities; or erectile disfunction.[99] In a 2017 review of penile enlargement surgeries, the researchers noted that the satisfaction rates of patients and their partners following this surgery were low, at 30–60%.[100]

Fat transfer injections have been one of the most popular and common cosmetic surgical options to increase penile girth.[101] Using liposuction, fat is harvested from another part of the body, usually the abdomen, thighs or pubic area. After the fat is purified, it is then injected under the skin of the penis (into the dartos layer) at four incision points evenly spaced around the penis. Once the fat has been injected, the penis is carefully kneaded to even out the fat deposits for a symmetrical and uniform finish.[102] This technique does have advantages – a patient's own tissue is less likely to be rejected, the incisions on the penis leave no visible scars, and the increased weight of the injected fat may contribute to some lengthening of the penis – and appears to have fairly good short-term results and patient satisfaction, with one study of 88 patients reporting an average girth increase of 2.65 cm after one year, and another reporting an increase of 2.71 cm after six months.[103]

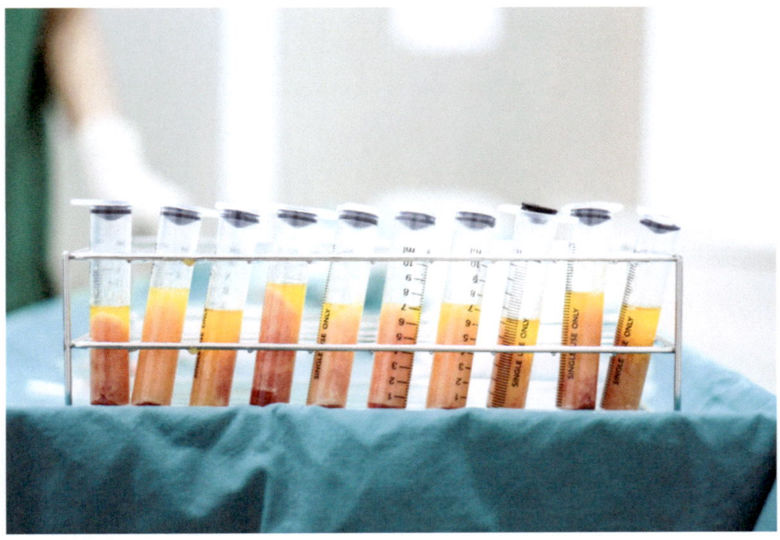

Harvested fat, ready to be purified and injected back into the body. (kpakook/ Shutterstock.com)

One problem with fat injections is that many of the fat cells may not survive the procedure (between 10–50%[104]), leading some practitioners to inject larger volumes of fat to compensate for this cell loss. However, larger volumes of fat have been linked to complications such as permanent nodules forming on the penis, curving, the loss of penile rigidity, severe deformities, or necrosis.[105] Injected fat is also likely to be reabsorbed into the body and may also be reabsorbed unpredictably, leading to a lumpy, uneven or asymmetrical penis.

Dermal fat grafts have also been used cosmetically for increasing girth. This procedure takes much longer and is more invasive than fat injections, with strips of fat surgically removed from elsewhere on the body, usually from the groin or buttock creases.[106] The fat is then surgically grafted under the skin of the penis through incisions at either the base or the head, either as strips, or as a sheet wrapped around the circumference of the penis. Dermal fat grafts can achieve a uniform girth increase of between 2 and 4 cm, but do come with the risk of severe complications and side effects. There might be large and unsightly scars where the graft was originally taken from; scar formation at the healing graft site may cause the penis to shorten or curve; and the graft tissue may not take or survive completely.[107]

Penile surgery for cosmetic purposes has a high risk for complications and unwanted outcomes, with low rates of satisfaction. During recovery following augmentation phalloplasty, it's necessary for patients to abstain from intense physical activity for a month, and all sexual activity (including masturbation) for between five and eight weeks and erections can be painful for a considerable length of time.[108] A scalpel approaching your penis is enough to put the fear of God into most people, even without the warnings from medical associations; a needle or cannula can be scary enough, but a more tolerable idea to many than surgery.

Injectables

If the thought of having your own fat injected into your penis makes you shudder, how would you feel about injecting something like paraffin or Vaseline? In the early 1900s, liquid paraffin and other mineral oils started being used as injectables to increase penis girth, but severe adverse effects were soon documented, including disfiguring nodules, ulcers, and skin necrosis, so these injections quickly fell out of favour with trained medical providers.[109] Despite these well-documented risks, liquid paraffin and mineral oils are still used today in the quest for a bigger penis, usually injected by non-medical personnel or self-injected by men themselves. Silicone, Vaseline, petroleum jelly, cod liver oil, palm oil, wax, and nandrolone decanoate (a type of anabolic steroid), or entirely unknown substances have been injected into penises over the years, with often devastating and irreversible consequences – including but not limited to allergic reactions, migration of the substance from the injection site, ongoing pain, ulcers, infection, tissue death, tumours, deformities, and sexual dysfunction.[110] While there's little statistical data on how many men around the world have these injections (including injecting themselves), studies suggest that it occurs more frequently in Asia and Eastern Europe – possibly as a result of the heavily patriarchal social structures in those communities.[111]

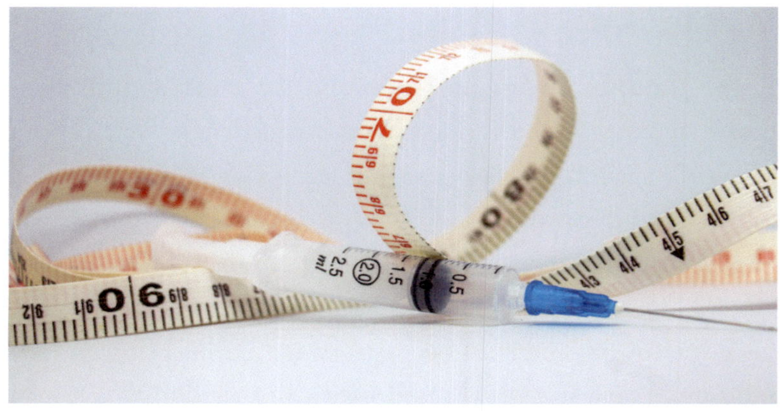

Injectables, despite their well-documented painful or dangerous side effects, have long been used by men in the search for bigger penises. (Viktor Valchyshevskyy/ Shutterstock.com)

A 2003 study of over 350 men in a Korean correctional institution who had had mineral oil injected into their penises found that many of them had done so because of a desire to appear more masculine before entering the prison system.[112] The vast majority (91%) of these men reported feeling unsatisfied with the results, with many experiencing inflammation, pain, difficulties with sexual activity as a result of the injection, and skin necrosis. A study of 680 men at a clinic on the Thailand-Myanmar boarder who had penile injections found that the majority experienced swelling and pain, including painful erections, and nearly half of them experienced severe complications, including hardening and disfigured penile skin.[113] There appears to be a large social element involved in these dangerous, medically-unapproved penis injections, with many men being introduced to or encouraged to undertake the procedure on the recommendation of friends or acquaintances[114] – to borrow a phrase, friends don't let friends ruin their penis.

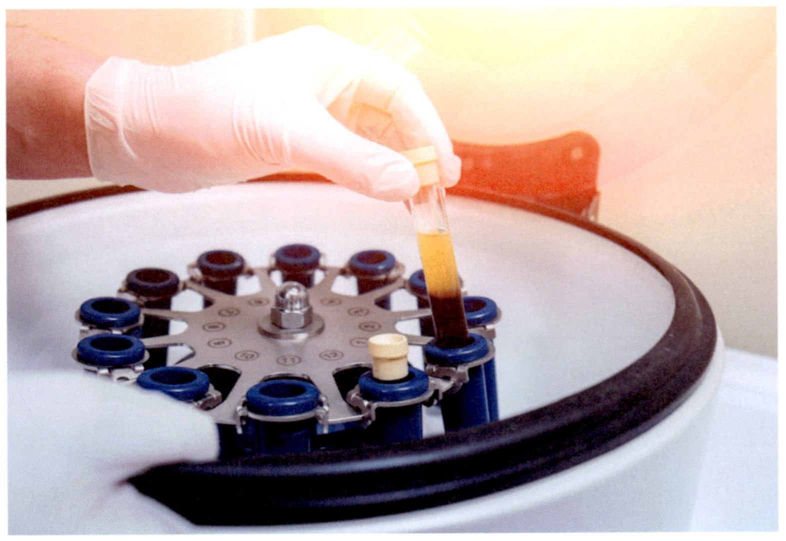

Blood is spun in a centrifuge to concentrate rejuvenating platelets, a type of blood cell, in plasma, the liquid portion of blood, ready for a platelet-rich plasma injection. (Roman Zaiets/Shutterstock.com)

Platelet-rich plasma (PRP) injections are an experimental treatment for erectile dysfunction, but some clinics advertise an increased penis size as an additional treatment outcome. Platelets are a type of blood cell which cause blood to clot, but they also contain growth factors which can stimulate tissue regeneration, healing, and cell reproduction. PRP therapy is used as a treatment all over the body for injuries and chronic pain; in tendons, ligaments, muscles and joints; as a way to accelerate healing after some surgeries; to treat hair loss, and as a 'vampire facial' treatment. To create PRP, a blood sample is taken from a patient and then spun down in a centrifuge to separate out other components in the blood and concentrate the platelets only within the plasma, the liquid portion of blood. This solution is then injected back into the patient's body, into the damaged or injured tissue that needs healing. The growth of new blood vessels following PRP injections into the penis, which is often advertised under the trademarked name 'the P-Shot', may potentially increase the volume of penis tissue slightly. However, while there is evidence that PRP may be an effective treatment for erectile dysfunction, there appears to be limited evidence that these injections offer any increase to penis size.[115]

Another interesting development is the use of muscle relaxants or anti-wrinkle injections as an alternative or adjunct to surgery and penile extenders. The penis and scrotum can contract involuntarily in reaction to cold temperatures or nervousness, due to the contraction of cremaster and dartos muscles. This phenomenon is colloquially called 'shrinkage'. When these muscles are overactive and contract without warning or reason, without the normal precipitant of nerves or cold temperature, this is called 'hyperactive retraction reflex'. The penis can then 'shrink' without warning or notice, which can at times be embarrassing for men. Injecting relaxants into the muscles which cause contraction and withdrawal of the penis and testicles can prevent this reflex. The muscle relaxant is injected superficially into the penis to relax the dartos muscle which contracts the penis, and also into the cremaster muscle which elevates and constricts the scrotum. It needs to be injected every three to six months and requires a significant amount of muscle relaxant, which can be prohibitively expensive. This procedure has humourously been called 'scrotox'. I have found this to be a relatively unsuccessful and expensive method of smoothing out wrinkles, and while there is some evidence that it might be useful in the treatment of erectile dysfunction, there is a risk that it might lower sperm count.[116]

Injectable dermal fillers have revolutionised cosmetic facial rejuvenation and surgery, and have held promise for penis enlargement as well. Since the 1970s, bovine collagen products have been used as injectable dermal fillers to plump out small wrinkles in the face, with success.[117] While there appears to be no scientific studies on the safety of bovine collagen for penis enlargement, it had been suggested as a viable option.[118] Its known qualities, however, make it a poor choice for penises. Bovine collagen products tend to be naturally reabsorbed by the body, sometimes lasting only three months, and they also have a relatively high rate of allergic reaction.[119] This means that patients would have to have regular collagen injections every few months, with significant risks of having a red, inflamed and lumpy penis if an allergic reaction were encountered.

Collagen biostimulators have also been popular as a facial treatment, and occasionally used in penises. When collagen biostimulators are injected into tissue, they create an inflammatory response which then stimulates the production of collagen and elastin. The new collagen and elastin create volume and plumpness in tissue.

One of these collagen biostimulators is a compound called poly-L-lactic acid, which is also found in the absorbable stitches used by doctors to close wounds. Poly-L-lactic acid is absorbable and temporary, with effects lasting up to three years.[120] Unlike other fillers, its effects are not immediate, but are delayed and gradual. One study into the efficacy and safety of poly-L-lactic acid for penile augmentation found that it did successfully increase girth, with participants gaining an average of 1.95 cm at six months, and that the results were maintained over time – at eighteen months, the average increase was measured at 1.79 cm.[121] The men in this study reported a significant increase in their level of satisfaction with the appearance of their penis after their treatment, but this level of satisfaction gradually decreased after around six months. However, they also reported a significant increase in their level of satisfaction with their sexual performance following treatment, and this satisfaction stayed consistently high eighteen months after treatment, even as their increased girth and satisfaction with their appearance both gradually decreased.

Despite these positive results, there are risks and complications involved. As poly-L-lactic acid is a foreign substance, it may cause an allergic reaction.[122] One well-documented risk of collagen biostimulators is that palpable and visible lumps can occur where too much stimulator is injected, or is injected too superficially.[123] Two studies of injectable poly-L-lactic acid into facial tissue found the risk of developing nodules and papules was around 7% and 9%, respectively, with most of these nodules and papules being described as mild to moderate and non-visible.[124] While small, palpable nodules in the face might not bother patients too much, it's easy to understand why palpable lumps in the penis might be undesirable, even suspicious. Incorrectly or inappropriately placed poly-L-lactic acid injections may also cause collagen overgrowth, which may be difficult to treat or correct as there is no simple way to reverse or dissolve poly-L-lactic acid once it has been injected.

Permanent dermal fillers also exist, but they are generally not recommended. As the saying goes, 'permanent fillers, permanent problems'. If you can't take them out when you have problems, everyone is unhappy. Permanent fillers which require no topping-up sound like a financial dream, but the problems can haunt you for a lifetime.

CASE STUDY

'Phil' recently came into my clinic to review his options. He had gotten permanent filler injected into his penis seven years ago on a trip to

Thailand, and in the last few years noticed that the filler had started to become lumpy. He had developed mobile nodules on the underside of his penis and also a firm, large, palpable lump at the base of his penis on the left side. While he did not want the nodules surgically removed, he decided to go ahead with hyaluronic acid dermal filler to try to minimise some of the irregularities. Phil was advised that the presence of permanent filler meant that he was at an increased risk for infections, but he elected to proceed with treatment. Due to the pre-existing irregularities caused by the permanent filler, it was a challenge to ensure a smooth application of filler, and we had to inject the last few milliliters of filler while Phil was standing up to ensure the best possible results.

The ideal filler would have a low rate of allergic reaction, be reversible, long lasting, inexpensive, and feel and look natural. Enter stage left, the penis enlarger for modern times: hyaluronic acid. Already used with great success to plump lips and cheeks, in experienced and sensible hands, hyaluronic acid dermal fillers fit the bill for penis enlargement quite well. Compared to previously used techniques it is overall the safest, quickest and easiest way to give a boost to penis size.

Hyaluronic acid filler

We all have approximately 15 grams of hyaluronic acid (or hyaluronan) in our own bodies.[125] It is a naturally occurring complex sugar which is part of the connective tissue scaffolding, or intercellular matrix, holding our cells together. It is found throughout the body, with the highest concentrations in joints, eyes, and skin. It has a natural affinity for water and can absorb a thousand times its weight in water, and it plays a major role in keeping skin hydrated and plump.

Hyaluronic acid has been approved for use as a dermal filler since the early 2000s, even in penises, and it has proved very popular for a few reasons. Injectable hyaluronic acid is nearly 100% bio-identical to that already in our bodies, which greatly reduces the risk of allergic reactions or rejection, estimated to be about 1 in every 1400 patients.[126] It is longer lasting with fewer complications than other fillers such as fat or collagen.[127] Hyaluronic acid fillers can also be reversed or corrected by injecting a dissolving agent called Hyalase, which is a purified preparation of an enzyme called hyaluronidase. Hyalase has been used to successfully dissolve hyaluronic acid filler even after five years.[128]

There are over two hundred hyaluronic acid preparations on the market which differ, sometimes significantly, in aspects of their formulation such as total hyaluronic acid concentration, molecular size, consistency, viscosity, and longevity.[129] Results following filler injections may vary depending on the formulation of hyaluronic acid, but high-quality, well-tested brands offer better results with far fewer complications.[130]

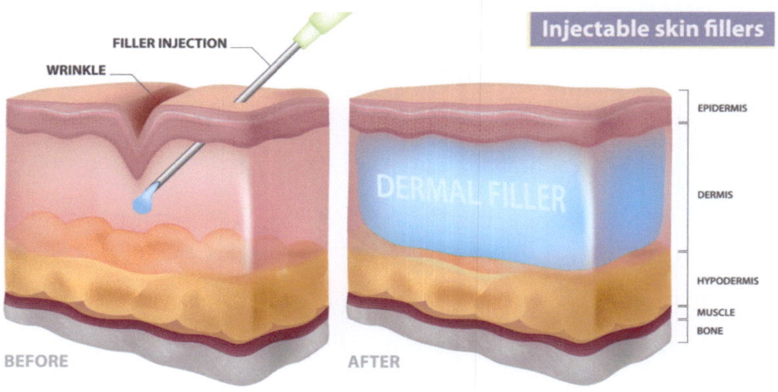

Hyaluronic acid is considered one of the safest, most popular, and long lasting dermal fillers. To plump out wrinkles, it is injected into the middle layer of skin. (Designincolor/Shuterstock.com)

The first documented use of hyaluronic acid in penises was to enlarge and shape the glans (the head of the penis) in the early 2000s.[131] In this study, only 2 ml of filler injected into the head of the penis increased its circumference by around 1.5 cm, a gain which remained steady a year after the injection.[132] Interestingly, this effect was still prominent in a follow-up study five years on, with an average decrease of circumference of only 15%. The good news from that study was that the men and their partners were as satisfied five years on as they were six months after their initial injections.[133]

It was only a matter of time before filler headed down the shaft to increase the size of more than just the head – with impressive results for that as well. One study found that injecting an average volume of 19.69 ml, participants' penis circumference had increased by an average of 2.2 cm six weeks following their treatment.[134] Another study found that with an average 20.5 ml injected, there was an average circumference increase of 3.9 cm after one month, which was maintained after eighteen months with only minimal loss (down to an average total gain of 3.78 cm).[135] While there were no serious adverse reactions reported in either study, either immediately following injection or in follow-ups, most patients reported a slight decrease in tactile sensitivity in the penile body.[136] This is because hyaluronic acid increases the connective tissue scaffolding between the skin and the internal nerve endings below, which reduces the sensitivity of the skin slightly. This slight drop in sensitivity was also reported when hyaluronic acid was only injected into the head of the penis, but the silver lining is that hyaluronic acid fillers may be a good treatment for premature ejaculation.[137] As a bonus, the weight of the fillers in the penis may also pull down on the penis's suspensory ligament, offering a slightly lengthening of 1–2 cm – similar gains to those offered by surgical lengthening, but much safer and less painful.

Some researchers note that the biggest limitation to using hyaluronic acid fillers for penis enlargement is finding a skilful enough nurse or doctor to inject it![138]

Tales from the Filler Doctor – What You Need to Know

As a GP and a cosmetic doctor, I've been injecting filler into almost every part of people's bodies for nearly twenty-five years. Filler has gone into cheeks and lips, but also necks to lift sagging skin, into ears to rejuvenate earlobes, to enlarge breasts and buttocks, into the backs of hands, even into people's feet to reduce pain. Penises were the next frontier for filler, and I started performing penis filler treatments around five years ago. It's growing in popularity, and I'm treating more and more clients. It's also become one of my favourite procedures to do because of the positive impact it has on my clients.

There have been challenges, though. There is a deeply puritanical streak in the world, which makes it very difficult to promote or advertise services affiliated with penis enhancement or augmentation. Facebook will knock back any posts even hinting at the word 'penis', and Microsoft's dictaphone program will not record the word in full, replacing the letters with asterisks.

But there are a lot of men out there who are interested in penis filler, and with some careful online and offline marketing and word-of-mouth, interested clients have been able to find their way to treatment. I get some questions quite frequently: about what actually happens during filler treatment, what kind of results filler really offers, and even about the type of clients I see. For all the details, read on.

What type of men get filler, anyway?

I must admit that I adore the men attached to the penises I fill. I find them to be mostly friendly, affable, interesting, successful men, and I love to hear their views on life. They're usually confident and know what they want, which makes them relaxed and easy to work with. Occasionally, cosmetic clients might be a bit on the high-maintenance side, but men coming for penis filler are rarely like that. This might be the opposite to what you would expect, but most men who enquire about penis filler have a penis that is within average size range. In my clinical experience, it is quite unusual for men who have smaller penises to enquire. Guys with smaller penises do occasionally pop in, but they are in the minority.

While the research suggests that some men who seek enlargement see themselves as small when they are not, in my experience, the majority of men who come to my clinic have a normal sized penis, *know* they have a normal size penis, and just simply want to have a larger one. Many men like a larger penis to boost their confidence and self-esteem, both in and out of the bedroom.

One lovely client of mine lived near the beach and simply wanted to feel comfortable doing what he loved doing, swimming and hanging around at the beach in his board-shorts and budgie-smugglers. Even though the increase in his size was not dramatic or even evident to others, it had a significant, deep and meaningful impact on his psyche. A moderate 20 ml of filler gave him a deep satisfaction that he was in the normal range and that people would not look at him sideways.

Wanting a larger penis, generally, seems to be related to the primal desire to win, to be superior, to be the alpha male at the top of the pecking order, the leader of the pack – and this attitude seems to be reflected in most of the men who come to my clinic. These men tend to be highly successful, at the top of their fields in business or industry. For these men, there is an element of excitement, a 'why not?' risk-taking attitude that serves them well in business. They're willing to try something new and adventurous. Why do these alpha male type guys get this done? Do they consciously think about a penis being a symbol of virility and fertility, being an expression of dominance in the herd? Of course not, but they are men pushing the frontier, wanting to be their personal best. One of my clients was largely retired by his early forties due to his prolific financial success; a dashing, handsome businessman, he came in saying, 'If I can't travel overseas because of COVID-19, what else am I going to spend my money on?'

Penis filler is a procedure which currently costs a lot of money, partly because so few doctors and nurses are skilled in the technique. While cheeks use approximately 2 ml of filler and costs around $1000, a good-sized penis filler takes 20 ml or more, which can cost $10,000 if using premium filler. To pursue having penis filler requires a modicum of financial success and comfort to start with.

Besides the financial winners-and-grinners, I also see a lot of men from the gym world – fitness fanatics and weight-lifters. These ultra-muscley men find that as their bodies have grown much larger, their penis now might seem a little out of proportion. If they have been taking body-building steroids, they may have even noticed that their testicles have shrunk. Usually, they are interested in bringing things back into proportion, and feel a larger penis complements their muscles more. Muscles are a status symbol in the gym or locker room, but a larger penis can be seen as one, as well. Filler allows these men to feel confident with their bodies, no matter where they are; it allows them to 'helicopter around' locker rooms with seemingly paradoxical nonchalance.

Another small subset of my clientele seeking penis filler treatments are the 'top dogs' of the underworld – men who are successful in their own unique way. These men tend to be a bit more reserved, a little less open, but they are still interesting men to treat. Their masculinity and their sexuality are worn like a badge of honour, and they are quite open about their sexuality and sex lives with one another. For some, their sexuality is almost a *raison d'être* – one of their main purposes in life, another way to be powerful. They do like to flout authority though, which can be a challenge. When we advise these men not to have sexual intercourse after the treatment to allow the filler to settle in, they usually laugh in a disparaging way, saying that would be unlikely to achieve. One of these clients disobeyed almost all of the post-care instructions: he took off his compression bandage after only half a day, rather than leaving it for the recommended three or four days; he had sex after three days instead of waiting at least one week. Luckily, and against all odds, he had an excellent outcome.

CASE STUDY

Bruce, 54, was a former military man who now owns a business. He is happily married with two children. His lovely and very supportive wife was completely happy with his current penis size. However, Bruce has wanted to increase his penis size since he was twenty years old, and believes the desire began when he was playing football and observed other men's penises when showering after games. He had a large cushion pad of fat burying his penis, but elected to have penis filler instead of a fat-removal procedure. He had given up on weight loss and didn't want to consider medications or surgical options for losing weight. Bruce was very happy with the results and plans to come back for another 20 ml.

It's definitely unusual for men to be motivated to get penis filler purely for the pleasure of their partner. Only one man I've treated claimed that this was his primary motivation. Most men seem to be motivated by wanting to improve their self-confidence and self-esteem, just for themselves. Often, they do it with no-one else knowing, sometimes not even their partner. About half of my clients don't tell their partners before their treatment, paradoxically hoping that they won't notice, but funnily enough, this is a pretty similar statistic to those getting facial cosmetic work. It might sound strange to think that a treatment like penis filler could go unnoticed by someone's intimate partner, but many people haven't heard of it, so they don't suspect it. One of my client's partners asked him about it, and he told her that he'd just been using an 'enhancing' moisturising cream. In my experience, though, most partners are quite supportive and encouraging, in a passive kind of way. They just want their partner to do whatever makes them happy.

Anatomy – where's the filler going?

Have you ever wondered why a penis doesn't get friction burns, rashes, or blisters during sexual intercourse? It is because there is a sliding space which moves back and forth during sexual intercourse to minimise friction. It is an inbuilt shock absorbing system where one layer of the penis can freely move upon another layer. The filler is injected between these two layers, called the dartos fascia and Buck's fascia. The filler can initially move around quite freely in this space, which is very expandable with its shock absorbing capabilities. It is like an inner and outer tube, similar to a tyre, and the space within can be pumped up with filler.

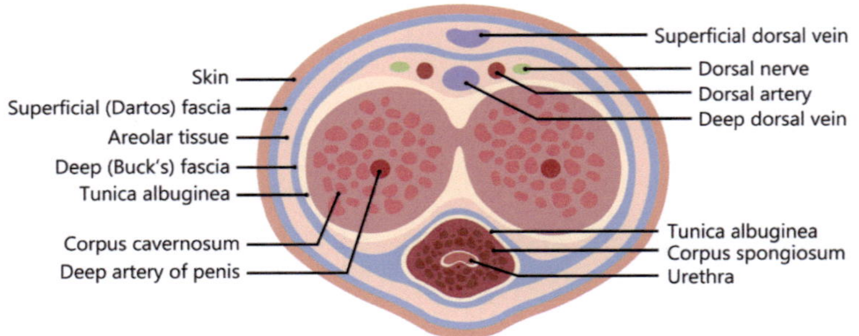

A cross-section of the anatomy of the penis. Filler is injected underneath the skin, into the areolar tissue between the dartos and Buck's fascia. (Kunteeg/ Shutterstock.com)

Having a foreskin can make the procedure more technically challenging. Ideally, filler should not enter the foreskin because it can inflate with its hydrophilic (water-absorbing) capabilities, creating lumps and bumps and giving a swollen look to the foreskin. Sometimes this can even create a deviation in the foreskin so it looks crooked, heading to one side.

If too much filler is placed in the foreskin, it can make it more difficult to retract the end of the foreskin. Some practitioners prefer not to inject uncircumcised men due to the higher need for revisions and tweaking afterwards.

Can I just have the head of my penis injected?

While overall size is important, so is keeping things in proportion – so if you're increasing the girth of the penis, it is a good idea to also increase the size of the head as well. This is more important for circumcised men where the head or glans of the penis is permanently on display. The conical glans or head of the penis is akin to the head of spear – a perfectly appropriate shape for vaginal or anal dilatation and entry. If the head is too large or too small for the shaft, the gliding intromission of the penis is impeded. The cushioning of the head or glans softens the thrusting of the tumescent corpora cavernosa, the two tubes of engorged blood responsible for the erection, and protects both the shaft of the penis and also the dome of the vagina.

Most guys would like a proportionate increase in the size of the shaft of the penis as well as the glans however there are some who just really want the head of the penis enlarged. Usually these are the guys who have been circumcised. If just the shaft is enlarged, the head of the penis may look relatively small and underwhelming.

The general rule of thumb is to use approximately a quarter or a fifth of the product in the head. The response of increase in volume is better in the shaft than it is in the head of the penis. The tension and lifting capacity is greater in the sliding space between the Buck's and the dartos fascia than in the more fibrous and 'tight' head of the penis. The head is an extension of the corpora spongiosum, the tissue which envelopes the urethra (the 'wee tube') and protects it. The maximum I have injected in the head in one sitting so far is 7 ml. The concern is that too much filler in the glans or head could cause too much swelling, which could temporarily obstruct the opening of the urethra and cause urinary retention and bladder distension, and then become a medical emergency.

The best bang for your buck with filler in the head of the penis is to insert it into the corona where the head of the penis meets the shaft. This can give the appearance of a 'frilly lizard in full bloom', but it is best to also extend and create a dome-like structure reinforcing the head of the penis.

It does take a significant volume of filler to produce a noticeable increase in size in the glans or head of the penis. Given the lower expandability of the more fibrous and dense head of the penis compared to the shaft, the satisfaction with enlargement of the head of the penis is not as high as it is with enlargement of the shaft of the penis. About half are happy with enlargement of the head while around 8 out of 10 guys are satisfied with enlargement of the shaft.

How is it injected?

This entire procedure takes about one to two hours. Firstly, the area is photographed from various angles – front, oblique and side on. The penis is then measured, taking the length from the peno-pubic angle to the end of the penis. The circumference of the penis is then measured at its widest part. These measurements are also photographed as well as documented. This can be the hardest part of the entire procedure – modesty has to fly out the window as doctors and nurses man-handle, measure and assess your penis. Once that is completed, everything else is easier.

Numbing cream is applied about half an hour before the procedure. Clients put this on themselves, and they often apply it liberally, thinking the procedure is going to be very painful. Most clients are often pleasantly surprised afterwards. Let's face it – the mere thought of someone bringing a needle anywhere near your penis is enough to bring tears to most men's eyes! But interestingly, this is one of the most comfortable treatments I perform. One of my clients who has had filler in his lips and muscle relaxant anti-wrinkle injections in his face said those procedures were much more painful than filler in his penis. He's so relaxed that he watches movies while he's being injected. Another client, a property developer, stays on the phone doing property deals, pretending he's in his office. Another client even fell asleep in the middle of the procedure!

The numbing cream helps a lot but occasionally a penile ring block, or local anaesthetic injection block, is performed at the base of the penis to numb the shaft. There is local anaesthetic in the filler as well so the whole process becomes more pleasant as you go along. We also offer inhalational pain relief, 'happy gas' or nitrous oxide, which makes it quite a relaxing and almost fun experience. Clients think we are quite excellent comedians while we are injecting because everything becomes quite amusing while under the influence!

After the numbing cream has been given time to work, it is wiped away and the area is thoroughly cleaned. Often, we inject clients with a medication called Caverject (alprostadil) to cause a semi or full erection. This gives a better definition of the area, and enables smoother application of the filler. Before Viagra was readily available, men experiencing erectile dysfunction would inject themselves with Caverject to achieve an erection in preparation for sexual intercourse.

Men often think that sharp needles are used during the procedure, however a blunt-tipped cannula is nearly always used to insert filler into the tissue. While some practitioners claim that needles give them more precision, cannulas are now the most popular choice. The beauty of the blunt-tipped cannula is that, under the guidance of a skilled operator, it gently pushes delicate nerves and blood vessels out of its path. Sharp needles, by comparison, slice and carve their way through tissue, causing more inflammation, bruising and swelling. A needle is needed to make a small hole for the cannula to be inserted into the penis – but apart from that, penis filler is almost a needle-free technique. After an insertion point is made with the needle, the cannula is inserted under the skin into the sliding space between the Buck's fascia and dartos fascia – that is, just under the skin. The cannula is gradually and slowly advanced along the sliding space in a parallel, oblique and transverse fashion to cover the entire shaft of the penis with filler in a uniform way, except for the underside of the penis, which is not readily seen.

The placement of insertion points is a contentious issue between practitioners. Some like placing one insertion point at the top front of the shaft, so they can manipulate filler around the shaft in a symmetrical fashion from that single injection site. However, others argue that this area is best avoided because of the dorsal penile artery and vein that run along the top of the shaft. Some practitioners prefer to create a single insertion site at the base of the penis near the pubic angle where the penis meets the stomach, or laterally on the shaft of the head of the penis where the foreskin remnants are attached (if the client is not circumcised, the insertion point is approximately where the foreskin inserts into the penis when the foreskin is retracted). Others prefer to insert filler from two or more sites spaced evenly around the circumference of the penis.

It really doesn't matter as long as the product is inserted in a smooth fashion; however, insertion of the needle can be the most painful part of the procedure, so the more puncture wounds there are, the more uncomfortable it may be for the client. Also, the more numerous the insertion points, the higher the risk of infection – even though the risk of infection with correctly-performed penis filler is very low. Fewer insertion points are also preferable, because occasionally, if the insertion site is slow to heal, filler can leak out. This is like molten gold escaping – filler is very expensive to buy, so any leakage is highly undesirable. Leaking filler can also cause lumpiness which will need to be corrected later.

After the injection, the penile shaft is thoroughly massaged to distribute the filler as smoothly as possible. An elastic compression bandage, often a self-adherent sports-type compression bandage, is applied for three to four days. Antibiotics are sometimes prescribed as well, particularly for immunocompromised clients such as those with diabetes.

Two weeks after the filler has been injected, the hyaluronic acid gel will have integrated into the penile tissue. Up until then, it might feel lumpy and irregular, as it does also in the lips and cheeks after injection. It takes about one month for filler to fully incorporate and integrate into the skin and three months for blood vessels to grow into the filler.

It is important to understand that this can be a two- or even three-step procedure and that a follow-up appointment is required one month after the first treatment to assess, revise and tweak the cosmetic result. Often, a bit more filler may have ended up at the head or at the base, or on one side or the other, and this will need a revision of up to 5 ml to smooth out. Penis filler needs more revision and tweaking than any other filler procedure in the body – and trust me, I have put it everywhere. You name it, it has gone there. When I first started doing penis enlargements, I thought these clients were just fussier than others, because after treatment they often requested 'a little extra in this area, more down there, more on this side, there's a lump near the top'. However, I have since realised penises can be quite tricky due to the 'moving feast' of filler in the sliding space. It is hard to control, reign in and anchor it in one place – unlike cheeks and lips where there is no 'sliding space' in which it can move around.

For this necessary purpose of tweaking and revising, it is important that clients understand that 5 ml will most likely be needed during the one month follow-up appointment. If he's committed to having 20 ml injected, then he must understand that he either has 15 ml injected at the first appointment and another 5 ml in a month's time, or he will need to purchase an additional 5 ml if he had the full 20 ml injected in the first treatment session. It is important the client understands this is not the fault of the injector, but is rather the 'nature of the beast'. They also need to understand this from a financial-planning perspective. Clients also need to understand the importance of aftercare in encouraging and maintaining the best outcome. That can sometimes be the hardest part of all – even more difficult than having the initial photographs taken!

How to look after it

Having filler is a big investment in yourself, so it is important to look after it. Hygiene is crucially important, but especially so in the first few days as the small insertion wounds are healing. The insertion wounds are often larger than those created when doing facial fillers, because a larger cannula is used when injecting the penis. On the face, it only takes up to six hours for the insertion wounds to heal over, however in the penis this can take one to two days because of the larger insertion hole and because the skin on the penis has a slower healing rate compared to the skin on the face. It's crucial to keep these insertion wounds clean while they are healing, to minimise the chance of any bacteria getting in and causing infection. A small, water-resistant bandaid is applied over the insertion points after the filler is injected, and should be kept in place for at least two days. There is no need to remove and replace it unless it falls off on its own accord, because removing it can cause the healing wound to tear open.

For one or two days following the procedure, you should wash your hands prior to touching your penis, including before you go to the toilet, not just after. Some doctors recommend using antiseptic hand washes for these first few days, but as long as the insertion sites are protected from contamination and you're using regular hand soap properly, that should be enough.

The biggest challenge in aftercare is maintaining the filler in the right place. Remember, the filler has been injected into the sliding space in between the superficial dartos fascia and the deeper Buck's fascia. Because this is a compartment where there is loose tissue, called 'areolar' tissue, filler can move around significantly within this space. It is unlike any other part of the body we might inject filler into, like cheeks or lips, where the filler is more tightly bound within the tissues and so can't move or migrate much, if at all. In the sliding space in the penis, the filler can be quite mobile.

Following the initial filler injection, a compression bandage is applied around the whole penis for three to four days to minimise swelling and to try and keep the filler in the right place. Bandages should not be too tight as to cause indentations in the shaft of the penis. Larger compression bandages are more desirable to minimise the edges carving indentations in the filler.

Clients should avoid heavy lifting or strenuous exercise for at least a week after their procedure, and abstain from sexual intercourse for at least one week to allow the filler to settle into place. Some doctors recommend abstaining from sexual intercourse for only two days while others recommend waiting at least a month, but one week seems to be the magical sweet spot, as the filler will have settled into position by then. Premature sexual intercourse will cause migration of the filler, squeezing the injected material distally and proximally. Sexual intercourse can push the filler more to the head because of the tightness at the opening of the penetrated orifice. If you have sex prematurely, your penis can be distorted – which can be alarming for men when they look down post-coitally! Sometimes filler can be massaged back into position but it can be hard work, so it's best just to avoid causing problems and wait.

It's best to avoid masturbating for the first two or three days following filler injections as well. Most men do not have much inclination for too much vigorous activity anyway, as they can feel quite tender and sore for a few days.

The movements of masturbation are quite similar to the massaging and moulding that is required to help the filler settle in place, which is why it's allowed so much earlier than sexual intercourse.

Vigilantly massaging and moulding the filler is crucial to getting a good outcome, mostly due to the stretchy sliding space that the filler is injected into. It takes about one week for the filler to 'set' into place, but the filler becomes increasingly difficult to move and work after about four to five days – so it's important to start moulding very early on in the process! Once the filler sets, if there are any lumps or bumps that haven't been massaged and moulded into a nice shape, the only option is to partially dissolve the filler by injecting a dissolving agent called Hyalase.

This moulding process is important because it helps to 'train' the filler to stay in the right place. It can ensure that the filler stays evenly distributed around your penis, ensuring that not too much goes to either the head or the base, and that you have a nice smooth appearance. I recommend that men massage and mould their filler for one minute each morning and night, as well as every time they go to the toilet. The penis should be massaged when both flaccid and erect, to ensure it looks good at all times. It can be easier and more effective to mould the filler during an erection though; not only is it more obvious where the filler is situated, but the erection offers some resistance to push the filler up against. When the penis is soft, there is less to push against so it can be more difficult to soften and mould the filler.

It's best to start moulding around three to four hours after the procedure. The massaging should be quite gentle on the first day to avoid causing any filler to leak out of the insertion holes before they've healed over, otherwise firm and strong massaging is required. Remember, the filler begins to set quite quickly and gets harder to move each day. Squeeze any smaller lumps and bumps vigorously between your fingers to help break them down. These are often located in the foreskin or near the head. It is better to keep the filler as much as possible on the top and sides of the penis, without moving too much of it to the underside, or ventral aspect, of the penis where it can't be visually appreciated as much.

After the treatment, the penis needs to be moved around into different positions so pressure (including from gravity) is exerted on it evenly. Remember the filler can slide around in the sliding space willy-nilly and we want it to set in the right place. The penis should not be left in one same position while filler is settling. If the penis is hanging down as it does naturally, with or without underwear, the filler can migrate down towards the foreskin, or towards the remnants of foreskin left by circumcision. This can create a ballooning effect near the head, or create some lumpy swellings. This has been referred to as a 'cricket ball in a sock' phenomenon.

Supportive underwear should be worn for at least a week to help keep the filler in place as it settles in and to minimise swelling. Supportive underwear helps ensure that the penis stays in place after its position has been changed – to the left and to the right, up and down, regularly moved around so that there is minimal repeated pressure on one particular area, which could create indentations or irregularities while the filler is settling in.

It is more common for men to have a deficit at the base of their penis with a ballooning effect in the middle or head, because they like to naturally let their penis hang down. Keeping it up and elevated in supportive underwear will minimise the risk of this happening. The impact of walking and running will also push the filler down towards the head if the penis is left hanging down without supportive underwear.

Penis extenders, vacuum pumps and peno-scrotal rings should not be used for at least one month so as not to cause uncontrollable shifts in filler.

Realistic expectations

Even the best civil engineer or mathematician would find it difficult to precisely predict the size increase that will be achieved by a given amount of filler, as the elasticity and expandability of tissue and skin can be quite variable between people, and the natural length of the penis will also have an impact on the possible increase in overall size.

As a rough rule of thumb, for a penis of average length, 10 ml of filler will add approximately 1.25 cm in girth or circumference to a flaccid penis, an increase of about 10%;

20 ml of filler will add around 2.5 cm in girth. Filler will increase the girth of an erection by approximately half of the flaccid increase on average, so 20 ml of filler will add approximately 1.3 cm to the girth of an erect penis.

While the increase filler provides is mainly in the girth of the penis, it may also increase the length somewhat because of the weight of the filler pulling down on the suspensory ligament of the penis. This can add a 1–2 cm increase in length when flaccid, but it will not increase the length of the penis during an erection. Interestingly, it appears most men are more concerned about the appearance and length of their penis when it is flaccid rather than when it is erect.

It is important to keep your expectations realistic, though. After filler has been injected, there will be some swelling which might take two to three weeks to go away entirely. When this subsides, it can be quite depressing for some. The swelling may make it look like you've had an extra quarter or a third of the actual filler volume you've had injected. For instance, if you've had 20 ml of filler, you may have about 25 ml-worth of filling *effect* until the swelling settles down. The mind often plays a mean psychological trick where people forget how they used to look and when the swelling settles down, they mistakenly think that the filler has all gone and can feel quite disappointed. This effect happens frequently in people who have had facial fillers too, so it's important for anyone getting filler anywhere to keep the swelling effect in mind.

Some men may have unrealistic expectations that penis filler will change their entire experience of life. They may expect potential partners to flock around them like moths to a flame. They may be disappointed that filler is not the secret ingredient to happiness they had been hoping for. The secret to happiness may not lie in a larger penis. The secret to good sexual and romantic relationships may not lie in a larger penis. This can be a disappointment to some. Studies suggest happiness depends on social interactions with others, a sense of belonging, a positive mindset, mindfulness, exercise and good health and a positive self-esteem.[139] A larger penis might help with a couple of those, but it is certainly not going to be the solution to all of your problems.

How big can you go?

When clients ask me, 'How much filler can be inserted in this space?', what I know they're really asking is, 'How big can I go?' Generally, I recommend men have 20 ml as an initial treatment. This gives enough oomph to be satisfied – as studies have shown – but then if they want more, they can always add more. This sounds like a lot, but 20 ml is only four teaspoons of filler. International recommendations suggest a maximum of 20 ml of filler in the face for women over the age of fifty, so 20 ml is not out of this world when it comes to the recommended dose for a penis. Imagine smearing four teaspoons of thick treacle around your penis shaft – it is not going to give a monstrously enlarged appearance at all, just a nice added layer. Some men chose to only have 10 ml due to budgetary constraints, but they tend to be underwhelmed, sometimes to the point of giving up and not returning for any more treatment. As Peta Autengruber, an Androfill injecting nurse in Adelaide, says 'It takes a few cans of paint to paint a house.' From experience, men who have 20 ml are more than twice as happy as men who have 10 ml. The beauty of the longevity of this procedure, though, is that you can build it up at any stage later on and add onto it.

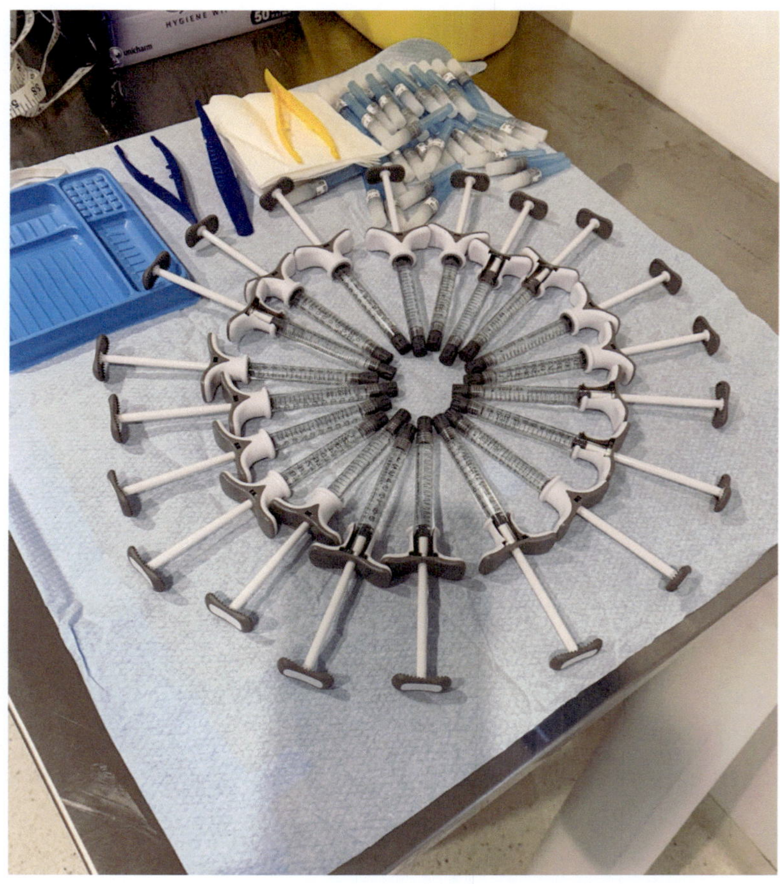

Syringes of hyaluronic filler, ready and waiting for the next client. (Courtesy of Dr Ingrid Tall, Androfill Brisbane)

The largest amount I have injected so far is 113 ml in total, but that client might have come back for a top up since the writing of this book! It can be addictive. His treatments have cost more than $50,000 Australian dollars in total, and nearly five years since his first treatment, he has reported absolutely no decline in the volume of his penis – so he considers the price worth it! He recently had another 13 ml injected, 7 ml of which went into the head of his penis to keep it in proportion. This client said he wanted to be his 'best self' and, like in his professional work where he is a very successful corporate executive, he simply wanted to push the frontiers. He appears to me to be a loving and monogamous family man, a wonderful father who succeeds also in work-life balance to spend time with his children. Another client of mine has had 70 ml in total injected into his penis. He told me he went to a 'naked disco' (I didn't know this was a thing) and that a young guy came up to him and said, 'You have the fattest cock I have ever seen, I just want to suck it.' A very successful outcome, in his books!

How long does it last?

Having covered the potential risks, the next big question is how long will it last? That depends, of course, which brand of filler you are using. Hyaluronic acid fillers are tempo-rary, and will slowly reabsorb into the body. Officially, shorter-acting fillers have a longevity of between six and twelve months, and yet the effect may last much longer.[140] I've been injecting for over two decades now and I continue to be rather astonished of the longevity of some of the more durable fillers. For example, the first two cheeks that I ever injected with durable, long-lasting filler are still present and effective well over ten years later. MRI scans have shown hyaluronic acid filler can be detected in facial tissue for as long as twelve years after it was injected.[141]

It is the same with penises. The first gentleman I injected, about five years ago, says it is still there 'one hundred per cent'. I have no reason to doubt his response, as studies have shown positive results after eighteen months, with one study finding that 85% of the hyaluronic acid filler injected into the head of the penis was still present even after five years.[142] Interestingly, the men in this study did not report noticing any visual reduction in size after five years, and their satisfaction levels remained consistently high, even as their added girth gradually decreased.

It is astonishing that filler can last so long, but the secret to its longevity may be due to its isovolemic degradation. As hyaluronic acid filler breaks down in the tissue, it is replaced with more water, and the gel volume balances itself out. It is thought there is increased water-binding capacity in the less concentrated hyaluronic matrix therefore it doesn't diminish in size.[143] Filler may break down more quickly in certain individuals, but this is rare. It is unclear exactly why this happens, but one hypothesis is that people with faster metabolisms may break down filler more quickly. People who are more physically active may metabolise their filler a little bit faster, as well.

What can go wrong?

The supportive underwear, the massaging and moulding, and the compression bandages are all designed to help the filler settle into the correct form, but despite all of these preventative measures, some men may require tweaks or revisions. One of the most common problems encountered is filler migration. I had one client who had a fastidious, pedantic personality. He wore a compression bandage religiously, didn't have sex for a whole month, and methodically changed the resting position of his penis so unequal pressure wouldn't be applied to any part. Despite this, he found he had some pooling of filler at the distal end of his penis near the head. Even if you do everything perfectly – massage vigorously for at least a week to even out the product, wear supportive underwear, minimise exercise, don't have sex, move the penis around into different positions, there can still be a need for tweaking and revision one month later.

It's important to understand that penis filler is usually a two- to three-stage process. About 8 out of 10 non-circumcised men desire a tweak or revision; and circumcised men are more likely to require a revision than non-circumcised. This is quite different to other filler procedures – rarely do people request a revision a month after getting filler in their cheeks! I revise less than 20% of clients usually, but with penis filler this is turned upside down and up to 80% will want a tweak done to smooth things out. This is not due to men being fussy and especially obsessive about their penises, it is simply about the mobility of the filler within the sliding space, which can lead it to be somewhat more unpredictable.

As a patient, it's important to articulate clearly what outcome you want with your penis so do not feel that you are being precious or especially demanding when you come back for your monthly check-up. This is part of the process. When you appreciate that this is a two- or three-stage procedure, it also allows you to financially plan your procedure.

One potential downside to penis filler is the problem of 'soft bone'. When more than 20 ml is inserted into the shaft, erections can feel slightly softer due to the thickness of the filler under the skin which covers the underlying corpora cavernosa, the two columns of spongy erectile tissue in your shaft that get hard during an erection. While this is not very significant with the first 20 ml, it becomes more noticeable thereafter. However, one client of mine who has had more than 100 ml injected has said that while he is aware of this, it doesn't bother him.

The filler may also absorb too much water and can occasionally feel a little soft or spongy. Sometimes during penetration, the penis can bulge a little at the base because of the pressure exerted by the tightness of the orifice. A little judicious use of Hyalase here and there can help correct this.

Another issue for some is that veins may become less visible or apparent in the superficial skin. While this isn't a downside in itself, it is important to realise that the visual look of your penis may change slightly, and may indicate that things are not as natural as they were before.

And a note for uncircumcised men: dermal skin filler can make it harder to retract your foreskin, which may make cleaning yourself more difficult. This is usually only a problem in men with previously tight foreskins. Dissolving a little of the filler in the distal foreskin can resolve this problem. Filler injections may also increase your risk of an acute medical condition called paraphimosis, where the foreskin becomes stuck in the retracted position behind the head of the penis. This can cause swelling, pain, impaired blood supply, and eventually tissue death. Paraphimosis may require urgent surgical release.

Are there any side effects?

Hyaluronic acid gel used for filler is very safe, and the risks are low, no matter where in the body filler is being placed. Even though problems do occur rarely, when they do happen they can be significant, and even catastrophic.

Bruising and swelling are some of the most common issues experienced with filler injections, but this is often mild and usually only occurs at the insertion point, rather than where the cannula is used. It is always best to reduce or stop taking aspirin, anti-inflammatories, fish oil, multi-vitamins, or ibuprofen for two weeks prior to the procedure to minimise the risk of bruising.[144] Swelling can be quite disconcerting in the first few days after the procedure. Your penis might feel especially boggy and soft, and the swelling might make it look almost deformed and indented occasionally. Most of the swelling settles down after the first few days but there is always a bit of swelling for around two to three weeks after.

Infection is a common potential complication following any surgical procedure, particularly if good hygiene practices aren't followed afterwards. However, in minimally invasive procedures such as filler injections, the incidence of infection is very low. In one study of 230 men who had undergone penile augmentation using hyaluronic acid filler, only two of them experienced infection – and both of those had pre-existing health conditions which made them more susceptible to infection.[145] In about a quarter of a century in practice, I have only seen one infection following hyaluronic acid gel filler injection, and that was in a patient's lips. I am aware of only one serious penile infection occurring in Australia following filler, where a penile abscess required surgical draining.

Another potential risk is of allergic reaction, but again this is a very low risk, estimated to be about 1 in every 1400 patients.[146] As hyaluronic acid is a substance found naturally in our own bodies, it very rarely triggers a rejection or allergic response, and most allergic reactions are thought to be caused by some kind of bacterial introduction, either during the manufacturing process of the filler or during post-procedure healing.[147] Immediate allergic reactions are usually very mild and resolve after a few days, with oral antihistamines effective at countering some of the symptoms; delayed allergic reactions may also resolve on their own, otherwise can be treated with oral steroids or by dissolving the filler.[148]

Vascular complications (that is, problems with the veins

or blood supply) caused by hyaluronic acid fillers are again very rare, estimated to be around 0.3%,[149] but they can be very serious. If filler is accidentally injected into a vein, or if a vein or blood vessel is constricted because too much filler has been injected into a very small areas, it can restrict blood flow and supply to tissue. This may cause scarring, ulceration, penile deformity or tissue death. In other words, parts or all of your penis could die and fall off! Luckily, vascular complications with filler are very uncommon. I have only seen one vascular complication in the head (or glans) of the penis in the more than five years I have been injecting penises, and despite it being hair-raising for both the client and myself, there were no significant long-term problems for the client.

Another complication of a filler procedure is iatrogenic priapism, in other words, a medically-induced erection that will not go down. Caverject is often injected into the penis to create an erection so filler can be injected more smoothly and evenly. This medically-induced erection usually goes down within an hour or so, but if it doesn't, it can be quite painful, cause blood supply to the penis to be impaired, and may require emergency medical treatment to prevent permanent damage. If the erection persists for more than a couple of hours, then a tablet or two of pseudoephedrine (Sudafed) can be taken, and if that doesn't work then medical help should be sought out quickly. I had one client who had an erection for nearly eight hours before it finally went down after he took some decongestant tablets. I rang a urologist for advice, who calmly told me I had to insert a wide-bore needle into the patient's penis and aspirate about 70 ml of blood. Luckily, things settled spontaneously (and with no long-lasting damage to the patient).

Conclusion

As a highly qualified working professional in this specialist area, I have tried to cover as many aspects of penis enhancement as possible. As history has shown, men have and will try many things in the quest for a bigger penis – including the incredibly dangerous – so it's important to be well informed about the safest, most painless, and most effective treatment.

Hyaluronic dermal filler for the penis is essentially a revolution in non-surgical penile enhancement. For whatever reason men choose to be part of this revolution, they can be confident in making a safe choice to enlarge their penis. With the latest medical advances in filler and filling technique, biology no longer has to be destiny, because your destiny can be what you choose to make it.

Unfortunately this choice was not available for the great Napoleon. When Napoleon died, the doctor who did his autopsy cut off his penis and gave it to a priest.[150] The penis did the rounds of private collectors and in 1977, it was finally bought by a New York urologist for $3000. It was valued at $1000 per half inch – meaning it was an inch and a half long in total. While the small, shrivelled, mummified object doesn't indicate how big Napoleon was when he was alive, it is tempting to wonder. Perhaps if Napoleon had been alive today, the current penis revolution could have changed the course of history. He could have made love, not war.

Endnotes

1. Chan, 'Cosmetic Surgery Statistics Australia and Around the World.'
2. Allergan, 'Allergan 360° Aesthetics Report.'
3. Krunik and Müller-Wille, 'Franz Boas and Inuktitut Terminology for Ice and Snow,' 377–400.
4. Allan and Burridge, *Euphemism and Dysphemism*, 96. Allan and Burridge also note that there are 'reportedly more than 1,200 terms for "vagina" and … 800 for "copulation"'.
5. Allan and Burridge, *Euphemism and Dysphemism*, 96.
6. Cormier and Jones, *The Domesticated Penis*, 88.
7. Angulo and García-Díez, 'Male Genital Representation in Paleolithic Art,' 12; Angulo, 'The Prehistoric Penis,' 61.
8. Angulo, García-Díez, and Martínez, 'Phallic Decoration in Paleolithic Art,' 2501–2; Angulo, 'The Prehistoric Penis,' 61.
9. Allen, *The Ancient Egyptian Pyramid Texts*, 168; Hart, *The Routledge Dictionary of Egyptian Gods and Goddesses*, 41; Cormier and Jones, *The Domesticated Penis*, 55.
10. Hart, *The Routledge Dictionary of Egyptian Gods and Goddesses*, 41.
11. Hart, *The Routledge Dictionary of Egyptian Gods and Goddesses*, 92.
12. Cormier and Jones, *The Domesticated Penis*, 58.
13. Neto et al., 'Gods Associated with Male Fertility and Virility,' 269.
14. Dasen, 'Probaskania,' 186.
15. McNiven, 'The Unheroic Penis: Otherness Exposed.'
16. Neto et al., 'Gods Associated with Male Fertility and Virility,' 270; Cormier and Jones, *The Domesticated Penis*, 68.
17. Cormier and Jones, *The Domesticated Penis*, 74.
18. Tagata Jinja, 'Hōnen Matsuri'; Cormier and Jones, *The Domesticated Penis*, 75.

19.   Cormier and Jones, *The Domesticated Penis*, 52.

20.   Cormier and Jones, *The Domesticated Penis*, 53.

21.   Cormier and Jones, *The Domesticated Penis*, 55.

22.   Lefebvre, *The Production of Space*, 98.

23.   Kennedy, *Transition*, 41.

24.   Cormier and Jones, *The Domesticated Penis*, 89.

25.   Fashion Encyclopedia, 'Penis Sheath.'

26.   Cormier and Jones, *The Domesticated Penis*, 100.

27.   Vicary, 'Visual Art as Social Data,' 8; Cormier and Jones, *The Domesticated Penis*, 101.

28.   Cormier and Jones, *The Domesticated Penis*, 101; Vicary, 'Visual Art as Social Data: The Renaissance Codpiece,' 8.

29.   Cormier and Jones, *The Domesticated Penis*, 102; Kosir, 'Modesty to Majesty.'

30.   Berlinger, 'How Gray Sweatpants Became the Unofficial Symbol of Fall Horniness.'

31.   Cormier and Jones, *The Domesticated Penis*, 18.

32.   Miller, 'Celebrity Bulges We Love'; Eliza Thompson, 'The 13 Best Superhero Bulges of All Time.'

33.   Norman, 'A man and his dog on a Sunday.'

34.   Greenstein, Dekalo, and Chen, 'Penile Size in Adult Men,' 153.

35.   King et al., 'Social Desirability and Young Men's Self-Reports of Penis Size,' 452, 454; King, 'Average-Size Erect Penis,' 84.

36.   Veale et al., 'Am I Normal? A Systematic Review,' 984; King et al., 'Social Desirability and Young Men's Self-Reports of Penis Size,' 81.

37.   Oates and Sharp, 'Nonsurgical Medical Penile Girth Augmentation,' 1033.

38.   Veale et al., 'Am I Normal? A Systematic Review,' 978.

39.   King, 'Average-Size Erect Penis,' 80; Johnston, McLellan, and McKinlay, '(Perceived) Size Really Does Matter,' 226.

40.   Grov, Parsons, and Bimbi, 'The Association Between Penis Size and Sexual Health Among Men Who Have Sex with Men,' 790.

41.   Lever, Frederick, and Peplau, 'Does Size Matter?' 134.

42.   Lever, Frederick, and Peplau, 'Does Size Matter?' 141.

43.   Shaeer and Shaeer, 'The Global Online Sexuality Survey (GOSS).'

44.   King, 'Average-Size Erect Penis,' 86.

45.   Wylie and Eardley, 'Penile Size and the "Small Penis Syndrome".'

46.   Pastoor and Gregory, 'Penile Size Dissatisfaction'; Johnston, McLellan, and McKinlay, '(Perceived) Size Really Does Matter,' 226.

47.   Pastoor and Gregory, 'Penile Size Dissatisfaction.'

48.   Oates and Sharp, 'Nonsurgical Medical Penile Girth Augmentation,' 1033; Lever, Frederick and Peplau, 'Does Size Matter?' 129.

49.   Panfilov, 'Augmentative Phalloplasty,' 185.

50. Veale et al., 'Sexual Functioning and Behavior of Men with Body Dysmorphic Disorder,' 153.

51. Choi et al., 'Second to Fourth Digit Ratio.'

52. Siminoski and Bain, 'The Relationships Among Height, Penile Length, and Foot Size.'

53. Shar and Christopher, 'Can Shoe Size Predict Penile Length?'

54. Greenstein, Dekalo, and Chen, 'Penile Size in Adult Men,' 155.

55. Orakwe and Ebuh, '"Oversized" Penile Length in the Black People: Myth or Reality'; Mondaini and Gontero, 'Idiopathic Short Penis: Myth or Reality?'

56. McGreal, 'The Pseudoscience of Race Differences in Penis Size.'

57. Veale et al., 'Am I Normal?' 983.

58. King et al., 'Social Desirability and Young Men's Self-Reports of Penis Size,' 83; Orakwe and Ebuh, '"Oversized" Penile Length In The Black People: Myth or Reality'; Mondaini and Gontero, 'Idiopathic Short Penis: Myth or Reality?'

59. Wylie and Eardley, 'Penile Size and the "Small Penis Syndrome".'

60. Cimador et al., 'The Inconspicuous Penis in Children,' 211.

61. Littara et al., 'Cosmetic Penile Enhancement Surgery,' 3.

62. Johnston, McLellan, and McKinlay, '(Perceived) Size Really Does Matter,' 227.

63. Lever, Frederick, and Peplau, 'Does Size Matter?' 139.

64. Francken et al., 'What Importance Do Women Attribute to the Size of the Penis?' 427–8.

65. Prause et al., 'Women's Preferences for Penis Size,' 3.

66. Prause et al., 'Women's Preferences for Penis Size,' 12.

67. Barnhart et al., 'Baseline Dimensions of the Human Vagina,' 1620; Worth, 'Does Vagina Size Matter?'

68. Psychologist Bernie Zilbergeld noted in his book *Male Sexuality* (23): 'It is not much of an exaggeration to say that penises in [men's] fantasyland come in only three sizes – large, gigantic, and so big you can barely get them through the doorway.'

69. Costa, Miller, and Brody, 'Women Who Prefer Longer Penises Are More Likely to Have Vaginal Orgasms (But Not Clitoral Orgasms),' 3083.

70. Shaeer et al., 'Female Orgasm and Overall Sexual Function and Habits,' 5.

71. Byers, 'The Interpersonal Exchange Model of Sexual Satisfaction,' 108.

72. Bergling, *Chasing Adonis*, under 'Parts is Parts'.

73. Haggas, 'Goldicocks.'

74. Drummond and Filiaut, 'The Long and Short of It,' 122.

75. Radkowsky, 'Is Size Everything in the Gay Dating/Hooking Scene?'

76. Ryan, Osborne, and Lowinger, 'Using Supplements?'

77. Corazza et al., 'Sexual Enhancement Products for Sale Online.'

78. Yuan et al., 'Vacuum Therapy in Erectile Dysfunction,' 211.

79. Yuan et al., 'Vacuum Therapy in Erectile Dysfunction,' 212; Min, 'Penile Traction Therapy (Penile Lengthening Device),' 162.

80. NHS, 'Penis Enlargement'; Fletcher, 'Penis Pumps and How to Use Them.'

81. Katz et al., 'Novel Extraction Technique to Remove a Penile Constriction Device,' 937.

82. Veale et al., 'Sexual Functioning and Behavior of Men with Body Dysmorphic Disorder,' 151; Martin, 'What Is Jelqing?'

83. Kim, 'History and Cultural Perspective,' 21.

84. Chung and Brock, 'Penile Traction Therapy,' 60–2; Campbell and Gillis, 'A Review of Penile Elongation Surgery,' 72.

85. Gontero et al., 'A Pilot Phase-II Prospective Study,' 794–5.

86. Nikoobakht et al., 'Effect of Penile-Extender Device,' 2188.

87. Dillon, Charma, and Honig, 'Penile Size and Penile Enlargement Surgery,' 519.

88. Marra et al., 'Systematic Review of Surgical and Nonsurgical Interventions,' 158; King, 'Average-Size Erect Penis,' 86; Oates and Sharp, 'Nonsurgical Medical Penile Girth Augmentation,' 1032.

89. Littara et al., 'Cosmetic Penile Enhancement Surgery,' 7.

90. Mayo Clinic, 'Penis-Enlargement Products: Do They Work?'

91. Urology Care Foundation, 'The Foundation's Recommendation on Penile Augmentation.'

92. King, 'Average-Size Erect Penis,' 84, 86; Campbell and Gillis, 'A Review of Penile Elongation Surgery,' 70.

93. King, 'Average-Size Erect Penis,' 86.

94. Campbell and Gillis, 'A Review of Penile Elongation Surgery,' 73; Chen et al., 'Visualization of Penile Suspensory Ligamentous System Based on Visible Human Data Sets,' 2437.

95. Campbell and Gillis, 'A Review of Penile Elongation Surgery,' 73; Alter, Salgado, and Chim, 'Aesthetic Surgery of the Male Genitalia,' 190.

96. Alter, Salgado, and Chim, 'Aesthetic Surgery of the Male Genitalia,' 190.

97. Dillon, Charma, and Honig, 'Penile Size and Penile Enlargement Surgery,' 524–5.

98. Dillon, Charma, and Honig, 'Penile Size and Penile Enlargement Surgery,' 525; Campbell and Gillis, 'A Review of Penile Elongation Surgery,' 73.

99. Dillon, Charma, and Honig, 'Penile Size and Penile Enlargement Surgery,' 525; Campbell and Gillis, 'A Review of Penile Elongation Surgery,' 73; Chen et al., 'Visualization of Penile Suspensory Ligamentous System Based on Visible Human Data Sets,' 2437.

100. Campbell and Gillis, 'A Review of Penile Elongation Surgery,' 73.

101. Dillon, Charma, and Honig, 'Penile Size and Penile Enlargement Surgery,' 523; Littara et al., 'Cosmetic Penile Enhancement Surgery,' 7.

102. Dillon, Charma, and Honig, 'Penile Size and Penile Enlargement Surgery,' 523; Littara et al., 'Cosmetic Penile Enhancement Surgery,' 5.

103. Oates and Sharp, 'Nonsurgical Medical Penile Girth Augmentation,' 1034.

104. Oates and Sharp, 'Nonsurgical Medical Penile Girth Augmentation,' 1034; Dillon, Charma, and Honig, 'Penile Size and Penile Enlargement Surgery,' 523.

105. Alter, Salgado, and Chim, 'Aesthetic Surgery of the Male Genitalia,' 190; Oates and Sharp, 'Nonsurgical Medical Penile Girth Augmentation,' 1034; Bizic and Djordjevic, 'Penile Enhancement Surgery,' 97.

106. Dillon, Charma, and Honig, 'Penile Size and Penile Enlargement Surgery,' 523.

107. Alter, Salgado, and Chim, 'Aesthetic Surgery of the Male Genitalia,' 190; Dillon, Charma, and Honig, 'Penile Size and Penile Enlargement Surgery,' 523–4; Campbell and Gillis, 'A Review of Penile Elongation Surgery,' 73.

108. Panfilov recommends five weeks ('Augmentative Phalloplasty,' 189), while Littara et al. recommend sixty days ('Cosmetic Penile Enhancement Surgery,' 7).

109. Bizic and Djordjevic, 'Penile Enhancement Surgery,' 97; Svensøy, Travers, and Osther, 'Complications of Penile Self-Injections,' 136; Ahmed et al., 'Self-Injection of Foreign Materials into the Penis,' e80.

110. Svensøy, Travers, and Osther, 'Complications of Penile Self-Injections,' 136. In his article 'The Shames of Men', anthropologist Don Kulick reported young men in Papua New Guinea injecting a mixture of 'baby oil and a white powder containing God-knows-what labelled *"Growim Kok"* (Penis Grower)'.

111. Svensøy, Travers, and Osther, 'Complications of Penile Self-Injections,' 136. Kulik, in his article 'The Shames of Men', noted that the motivation in the cases he observed in Papua New Guinea was that a 'big penis … was a means of controlling women.'

112. Moon et al., 'Sexual Function and Psychological Characteristics of Penile Paraffinoma.' Interestingly, 22% of these men reported that a qualified medical practitioner had performed the injection.

113. Svensøy, Travers, and Osther, 'Complications of Penile Self-Injections,' 139.

114. Svensøy, Travers, and Osther, 'Complications of Penile Self-Injections,' 141; Moon et al., 'Sexual Function and Psychological Characteristics of Penile Paraffinoma'; Rosecker et al., 'Hungarian "Jailhouse Rock"'; Kulik, 'The Shames of Men.'

115. Poulios et al., 'Platelet-Rich Plasma (PRP) Improves Erectile Function'; Epifanova, 'Platelet-Rich Plasma Therapy for Male Sexual Dysfunction.'

116. Jewell, 'Scrotox: Does It Work?'

117. Kim et al., 'Long-Term Safety and Longevity of a Mixture of Polymethyl Methacrylate and Cross-Linked Dextran (Lipen-10®) after Penile Augmentation,' 203.

118. Yang, Lee, and Kim, 'Tolerability and Efficacy of Newly Developed Penile Injection of Cross-Linked Dextran and Polymethylmethacrylate Mixture on Penile Enhancement'; Elist, 'Penile Enlargement Filler Facts.'

119. Kim et al., 'Long-Term Safety and Longevity of a Mixture of Polymethyl Methacrylate and Cross-Linked Dextran (Lipen-10®) after Penile Augmentation,' 203.

120. Sickles, Nassereddin, and Gross, *Poly-L-Lactic Acid*; Yang et al., 'Comparison of Clinical Outcomes between Hyaluronic and Polylactic Acid Filler Injections for Penile Augmentation in Men Reporting a Small Penis,' 1024.

121. Yang et al., 'Comparison of Clinical Outcomes between Hyaluronic and Polylactic Acid Filler Injections for Penile Augmentation in Men Reporting a Small Penis,' 1024.

122. Sickles, Nassereddin, and Gross, *Poly-L-Lactic Acid.*

123. Sickles, Nassereddin, and Gross, *Poly-L-Lactic Acid.*

124. Bauer and Graivier, 'Optimizing Injectable Poly-L-Lactic Acid Administration for Soft Tissue Augmentation,' e26; Narins et al., 'A Randomized Study of the Efficacy and Safety of Injectable Poly-L-Lactic Acid,' 459.

125. Stern, 'Hyaluronan Catabolism,' 317.

126. Abduljabbar and Basendwh, 'Complications of Hyaluronic Acid Fillers and Their Managements,' 102.

127. Tae Ahn et al., 'Efficacy and Safety of Penile Girth Enhancement Using Hyaluronic Acid Filler,' 2; Abduljabbar and Basendwh, 'Complications of Hyaluronic Acid Fillers and Their Managements,' 101.

128. King, Convery, and Davies, 'The Use of Hyaluronidase in Aesthetic Practice (v2.4),' e62.

129. Haneke, 'Managing Complications of Fillers,' 200, 201; Abduljabbar and Basendwh, 'Complications of Hyaluronic Acid Fillers and Their Managements,' 102.

130. Haneke, 'Managing Complications of Fillers,' 200.

131. Kim et al., 'Human Glans Penis Augmentation Using Injectable Hyaluronic Acid Gel'; Bizic and Djordjevic, 'Penile Enhancement Surgery,' 98.

132. Kim et al., 'Human Glans Penis Augmentation Using Injectable Hyaluronic Acid Gel,' 440.

133. Kwak et al., 'Long-Term Effects of Glans Penis Augmentation Using Injectable Hyaluronic Acid Gel for Premature Ejaculation,' 426.

134. Tae Ahn et al., 'Efficacy and Safety of Penile Girth Enhancement Using Hyaluronic Acid Filler,' 4.

135. Kwak et al., 'The Effects of Penile Girth Enhancement Using Injectable Hyaluronic Acid Gel, a Filler,' 3409–10.

136. Kwak et al., 'The Effects of Penile Girth Enhancement Using Injectable Hyaluronic Acid Gel, a Filler,' 3411.

137. Kwak et al., 'Long-Term Effects of Glans Penis Augmentation Using Injectable Hyaluronic Acid Gel for Premature Ejaculation,' 427.

138. Kwak et al., 'The Effects of Penile Girth Enhancement Using Injectable Hyaluronic Acid Gel, a Filler,' 3411.

139. Medvedev and Landhuis, 'Exploring Constructs of Well-Being, Happiness and Quality of Life,' 2–5.

140. Haneke, 'Managing Complications of Fillers,' 201; Quan et al., 'Complications and Management of Penile Augmentation with Hyaluronic Acid Injection,' 393.

141. Master, 'Hyaluronic Acid Filler Longevity and Localization,' 50e.

142. Kwak et al., 'Long-Term Effects of Glans Penis Augmentation Using Injectable Hyaluronic Acid Gel for Premature Ejaculation,' 426.

143. Kwak et al., 'Long-Term Effects of Glans Penis Augmentation Using Injectable Hyaluronic Acid Gel for Premature Ejaculation,' 427.

144. Abduljabbar and Basendwh, 'Complications of Hyaluronic Acid Fillers and Their Managements,' 101.

145. Quan et al., 'Complications and Management of Penile Augmentation with Hyaluronic Acid Injection,' 394.

146. Abduljabbar and Basendwh, 'Complications of Hyaluronic Acid Fillers and Their Managements,' 102.

147. Quan et al., 'Complications and Management of Penile Augmentation with Hyaluronic Acid Injection,' 393; Barmettler and Thuma, 'Complications of Hyaluronic Acid Fillers,' under 'Allergic Reactions'.

148. Barmettler and Thuma, 'Complications of Hyaluronic Acid Fillers,' under 'Allergic Reactions'.

149. Barmettler and Thuma, 'Complications of Hyaluronic Acid Fillers,' under 'Vascular Complications'. Last modified November 17, 2021.

150. Kirti, 'The Bizarre Journey of Napoleon Bonaparte's Penis.'

Bibliography

Abduljabbar, Mohammed H., and Mohammad A. Basendwh. 'Complications of Hyaluronic Acid Fillers and Their Managements,' *Journal of Dermatology & Dermatologic Surgery* 20 (2016): 100–106.

Ahmed, Usama, Alex Freeman, A. Kirkham, D. J. Ralph, S. Minhas, and Asif Muneer. 'Self-Injection of Foreign Materials into the Penis.' *Annals of the Royal College of Surgeons of England* 99, no. 2 (2017): e78–e82.

Allan, Keith, and Kate Burridge. *Euphemism and Dysphemism: Language Used As Shield and Weapon.* New York: Oxford University Press, 1991.

Allen, James P. *The Ancient Egyptian Pyramid Texts.* 2nd ed. Atlanta: Society of Biblical Literature Press, 2015.

Allergan. 'Allergan 360° Aesthetics Report – 2019 Edition.' Accessed November 1, 2021. https://www.allergan.com/medical-aesthetics/allergan-360-aesthetics-report.

Alter, Gary, Christopher Salgado, and Harvey Chim. 'Aesthetic Surgery of the Male Genitalia.' *Seminars in Plastic Surgery* 25, no. 3 (August 2011): 189–195.

Angulo, Javier C., and Marcos García-Díez. 'Male Genital Representation in Paleolithic Art: Erection and Circumcision Before History.' *Urology* 74, no. 1 (July 2009): 10–14.

Angulo, Javier. 'The Prehistoric Penis.' *EMJ Urology* 4, no. 1 (April 2016): 60–61.

Angulo, Javier C., Marcos García-Díez, and Marc Martínez. 'Phallic Decoration in Paleolithic Art: Genital Scarification, Piercing and Tattoos.' *The Journal of Urology* 186, no. 6 (December 2011): 2498–2503.

Barnhart, Kurt T., Adriana Izquierdo, E. Scott Pretorius, David M. Shera, Mayadah Shabbout, and Alka Shaunik. 'Baseline Dimensions of the Human Vagina.' *Human Reproduction* 21, no. 6 (2006): 1618–1622.

Bauer, Ute, and Miles H. Graivier. 'Optimizing Injectable Poly-L-Lactic Acid

Administration for Soft Tissue Augmentation: The Rationale for Three Treatment Sessions.' *Canadian Journal of Plastic Surgery* 19, no. 3 (2011): e22-e27.

Bergling, Tim. *Chasing Adonis: Gay Men and the Pursuit of Perfection.* New York: Taylor & Francis, 2013.

Berlinger, Max. 'How Gray Sweatpants Became the Unofficial Symbol of Fall Horniness.' *GQ,* September 28, 2020. https://www.gq.com/story/grey-sweatpants-meme-explained.

Barmettler, Anne, And Tobin Thuma. 'Complications of Hyaluronic Acid Fillers.' EyeWiki: American Academy of Ophthalmology. https://eyewiki.aao.org/Complications_of_Hyaluronic_Acid_Fillers.

Bizic, Marta R., and Miroslav L. Djordjevic. 'Penile Enhancement Surgery: An Overview.' *European Medical Journal* 4, no. 1 (April 2016): 94–100.

Byers, E. Sandra. 'The Interpersonal Exchange Model of Sexual Satisfaction: Implications for Sex Therapy with Couples.' *Canadian Journal of Counselling* 33, no. 2 (1999): 95–111.

Campbell, Jeffrey, and Joshua Gillis. 'A Review of Penile Elongation Surgery.' *Translational Andrology and Urology* 6, no. 1 (February 2017): 69–78.

Chan, Gavin. 'Cosmetic Surgery Statistics Australia and Around the World.' Victorian Cosmetic Institute. Last modified January 16, 2020. https://www.thevictoriancosmeticinstitute.com.au/2020/01/cosmetic-surgery-statistics-australia-around-the-world.

Chen, Xianzhuo, Yi Wu, Ling Tao, Yan Yan, Jun Pang, Shaoxiang Zhang, and Shirong Li. 'Visualization of Penile Suspensory Ligamentous System Based on Visible Human Data Sets.' *Medical Science Monitor* 23 (2017): 2436–2444.

Choi, In Ho, Khae Hawn Kim, Han Jung, Sang Jin Yoon, Soo Woong Kim, and Tae Beom Kim. 'Second to Fourth Digit Ratio: A Predictor of Adult Penile Length.' *Asian Journal of Andrology* 13, no. 5 (September 2011): 710–714.

Chung, Eric, and Gerald Brock. 'Penile Traction Therapy and Peyronie's Disease: A State of Art Review of the Current Literature.' *Theraputic Advances in Urology* 5, no. 1 (2013): 59–65.

Cimador, Marcello, Pieralba Catalano, Rita Ortolano and Mario Giuffrè. 'The Inconspicuous Penis in Children.' *Nature Review Urology* 12 (2015): 205–215.

Cormier, Loretta A., and Sharyn R. Jones. *The Domesticated Penis: How Womanhood Has Shaped Manhood.* Tuscaloosa: The University of Alabama Press, 2015.

Corazza, Ornella, Giovanni Martinotti, Rita Santacroce, Eleonora Chillemi, Massimo Di Giannantonio, Fabrizio Schifano, and Selim Cellek. 'Sexual Enhancement Products for Sale Online: Raising Awareness of the Psychoactive Effects of Yohimbine, Maca, Horny Goat Weed, and Ginkgo Biloba.' *BioMed Research International* 5 (June 2014): e841798.

Costa, Rui Miguel, Geoffrey F. Miller, and Stuart Brody. 'Women Who Prefer

Longer Penises Are More Likely to Have Vaginal Orgasms (But Not Clitoral Orgasms): Implications for an Evolutionary Theory of Vaginal Orgasm.' *Journal of Sexual Medicine* 9, no. 12 (December 2012): 3079–3088.

Dasen, Véronique. 'Probaskania: Amulets and Magic in Antiquity.' In *The Materiality of Magic*, edited by Dietrich Boschung and Jan N. Bremmer, 177–204. Paderborn: Wilhelm Fink, 2015.

Dillon, B. E., N. B. Charma, and S. C. Honig. 'Penile Size and Penile Enlargement Surgery: A Review.' *International Journal of Impotence Research* 20 (2008): 519–529.

Drummond, Murray J. N., and Shaun M. Filiault. 'The Long and Short of It: Gay Men's Perceptions of Penis Size.' *Gay and Lesbian Issues and Psychology Review* 3, no. 2 (January 2007): 121–9.

Elist, James. 'Penile Enlargement Filler Facts.' Accessed November 1, 2021. https://www.drelist.com/patient-education/myths-and-facts/fillers-facts.

Epifanova, Maya V., Badri R. Gvasalia, Maksim A. Durashov, Sergey A. Artemenko. 'Platelet-Rich Plasma Therapy for Male Sexual Dysfunction: Myth or Reality?' *Sexual Medicine Reviews* 8, no. 1 (January 2020): 106–113.

Fashion Encyclopedia. 'Penis Sheath.' Accessed November 24, 2021. http://www.fashionencyclopedia.com/fashion_costume_culture/The-Ancient-World-Egypt/Penis-Sheath.html.

Fletcher, Jenna. 'Penis Pumps and How to Use Them.' Medical News Today. Last modified September 19, 2019. https://www.medicalnewstoday.com/articles/326394.

Francken, A. B., H. B. M van de Wiel, M. F. van Driel, and W. C. M. Weijmar Schultz, 'What Importance Do Women Attribute to the Size of the Penis?' *European Urology* 42 (2002): 426–431.

Gontero, Paolo, Massimiliano Di Marco, Gianluca Giubilei, Riccardo Bartoletti, Giovanni Pappagallo, Alessandro Tizzani, and Nicola Mondaini. 'A Pilot Phase-II Prospective Study to Test the "Efficacy" and Tolerability of a Penile-Extender Device in the Treatment of "Short Penis".' *BJU International* 103, no. 6 (March 2009): 793–797.

Greenstein, Alexander, Snir Dekalo, and Juza Chen. 'Penile Size in Adult Men – Recommendations for Clinical and Research Measurements.' *International Journal of Impotence Research* 32, no. 2 (2020): 153–158.

Grov, Christian, Jeffrey T. Parsons, and David S. Bimbi. 'The Association Between Penis Size and Sexual Health Among Men Who Have Sex with Men.' *Archives of Sexual Behavior* 39 (2010): 788–797.

Haggas, Stuart, 'Goldicocks: The Penis Issue.' LGBT Hero. Accessed November 24, 2021. https://www.lgbthero.org.uk/fs160-the-penis-issue.

Haneke, Eckart. 'Managing Complications of Fillers: Rare and Not-So Rare.' *Journal of Cutaneous and Aesthetic Surgery* 8, no. 4 (2015): 198-210.

Hart, George. *The Routledge Dictionary of Egyptian Gods and Goddesses.* 2nd ed. New York: Routledge, 2005.

Jewell, Tim. 'Scrotox: Does It Work?' Healthline. Last modified May 28, 2019. https://www.healthline.com/health/scrotox.

Johnston, Lucy, Tracey McLellan, and Audrey McKinlay. '(Perceived) Size Really Does Matter: Male Dissatisfaction with Penis Size.' *Psychology of Men & Masculinity* 15, no. 2 (2014): 225–228.

Katz, Darren J., Warren Chin, Sree Appu, Matthew Harper, Filip Vukasin, Yeng Kwang Tay, Chia Pang, and Caroline Dowling. 'Novel Extraction Technique to Remove a Penile Constriction Device.' *Journal of Sexual Medicine* 9, no. 3 (March 2012): 937–940.

Kennedy, Margrit. *Transition.* Michigan: University of Michigan Press, 1988.

Kim, J. J., T. I. Kwak, B. G. Jeon, J. Cheon, and D. G. Moon. 'Human Glans Penis Augmentation Using Injectable Hyaluronic Acid Gel.' *International Journal of Impotence Research* 15 (2003): 439–443.

Kim, Ma Tae, Kyungtae Ko, Won Ki Lee, Sae Chul Kim, and Dae Yul Yang. 'Long-Term Safety and Longevity of a Mixture of Polymethyl Methacrylate and Cross-Linked Dextran (Lipen-10®) after Penile Augmentation: Extension Study from Six to 18 Months of Follow-Up.' *World Journal of Men's Health* 33, no. 3 (December 2015): 202–208.

Kim, Won Whe. 'History and Cultural Perspective.' In *Penile Augmentation*, edited by Nam Cheol Park, Sae Woong Kim, and Du Geon Moon, 11–26. Berlin: Springer, 2016.

King, Bruce M. 'Average-Size Erect Penis: Fiction, Fact, and the Need for Counseling.' *Journal of Sex & Marital Therapy* 47, no. 1 (2021): 80–89.

King, Bruce M., Lauren M. Duncan, Kelley M. Clinkenbeard, Morgan B. Rutland, and Kelly M. Ryan. 'Social Desirability and Young Men's Self-Reports of Penis Size.' *Journal of Sex & Marital Therapy* 45, no. 5 (2019): 452–455.

King, Martyn, Cormac Convery, and Emma Davies. 'The Use of Hyaluronidase in Aesthetic Practice (v2.4).' *Journal of Clinical and Aesthetic Dermatology* 11, no. 6 (June 2018): e61-e68.

Kirti, Kamna. 'The Bizarre Journey of Napoleon Bonaparte's Penis.' Medium. Last modified August 30, 2020. https://medium.com/the-collector/the-bizarre-journey-of-napoleon-bonapartes-penis-a18fcfce8780.

Kosir, Beth Marie. 'Modesty to Majesty: The Development of the Codpiece.' Richard III Society. Accessed November 24, 2021. http://www.r3.org/richard-iii/15th-century-life/15th-century-life-articles/modesty-to-majesty-the-development-of-the-codpiece.

Krupnik, Igor, and Ludger Müller-Wille. 'Franz Boas and Inuktitut Terminology for Ice and Snow: From the Emergence of the Field to the "Great Eskimo

Vocabulary Hoax".' In *SIKU: Knowing Our Ice*, edited by Igor Krupnik, Claudio Aporta, Shari Gearheard, Gita J. Laidler, and Lene Kielsen Holm, 377–400. Dordrecht: Springer, 2010.

Kulick, Don. 'The Shames of Men.' Longreads. Last modified June 6, 2019. https://longreads.com/2019/06/26/the-shames-of-men.

Kwak, T. I., M. H. Jin, J. J. Kim, and D. G. Moon. 'Long-Term Effects of Glans Penis Augmentation Using Injectable Hyaluronic Acid Gel for Premature Ejaculation.' *International Journal of Impotence Research* 20 (2008): 425–428.

Kwak, Tae Il, MiMi Oh, Je Jong Kim, and Du Geon Moon. 'The Effects of Penile Girth Enhancement Using Injectable Hyaluronic Acid Gel, a Filler.' *Journal of Sexual Medicine* 8 (2011): 3407–3413.

Lefebvre, Henri. *The Production of Space.* Malden: Blackwell Publishing, 2009.

Lever, Janet, David A. Frederick, and Letitia Anne Peplau. 'Does Size Matter? Men's and Women's Views on Penis Size Across the Lifespan.' *Psychology of Men & Masculinity* 7, no. 3 (2006): 129–143.

Littara, Alessandro, Roberto Melone, Julio Cesar Morales-Medina, Tommaso Iannitti, and Beniamino Palmieri. 'Cosmetic Penile Enhancement Surgery: A 3-Year Single-Centre Retrospective Clinical Evaluation of 355 Cases.' *Scientific Reports* 9, article no. 6323 (2019).

Marra, Giancarlo, Andrew Drury, Lisa Tran, David Veale, Gordon H. Muir. 'Systematic Review of Surgical and Nonsurgical Interventions in Normal Men Complaining of Small Penis Size.' *Sexual Medicine Reviews* 8, no. 1 (January 2020): 158-180.

Martin, Michael. 'What Is Jelqing? Will It Make My Penis Bigger?' RO Health Guide. Last modified November 16, 2021. https://ro.co/health-guide/what-is-jelqing.

Master, Mobin. 'Hyaluronic Acid Filler Longevity and Localization: Magnetic Resonance Imaging Evidence.' *Plastic and Reconstructive Surgery* 147, no. 1 (January 2021): 50e-53e.

Mayo Clinic. 'Penis-Enlargement Products: Do They Work?' Last modified June 3, 2020. https://www.mayoclinic.org/healthy-lifestyle/sexual-health/in-depth/penis/art-20045363.

McGreal, Scott A. 'The Pseudoscience of Race Differences in Penis Size.' Psychology Today. Last modified October 16, 2012. https://www.psychology today.com/au/blog/unique-everybody-else/201210/the-pseudoscience-race-differences-in-penis-size.

McNiven, Timothy J. 'The Unheroic Penis: Otherness Exposed.' *Notes in the History of Art* 15, no. 1 (1995): 10-16.

Medvedev, Oleg N., and C. Erik Landhuis. 'Exploring Constructs of Well-Being, Happiness and Quality of Life.' *PeerJ* 6 (2018): e4903.

Miller, Korin. 'Celebrity Bulges We Love.' *Cosmopolitan*, September 20, 2012. https://www.cosmopolitan.com/entertainment/celebs/news/g2255/celebrity-bulges.

Min, Kweon Sik. 'Penile Traction Therapy (Penile Lengthening Device).' In *Penile Augmentation*, edited by Nam Cheol Park, Sae Woong Kim, and Du Geon Moon, 159–168. Berlin: Springer, 2016.

Mondaini, Nicola, and Paolo Gontero. 'Idiopathic Short Penis: Myth or Reality?' *BJU International* 95, no. 1 (2005): 8–9.

Moon, Du Geon, Jeong Woo Yoo, Jae Hyun Bae, Chang Su Han, Yong Ku Kim, and Je Jong Kim. 'Sexual Function and Psychological Characteristics of Penile Paraffinoma.' *Asian Journal of Andrology* 5, no. 3 (September 2003): 191–194.

Narins, Rhoda S., Leslie Baumann, Fredric S. Brandt, Steven Fagien, Scott Glazer, Nicholas J. Lowe, Gary D. Monheit, Marta I. Rendon, Rod J. Rohrich, and Philip Werschler. 'A Randomized Study of the Efficacy and Safety of Injectable Poly-L-Lactic Acid versus Human-Based Collagen Implant in the Treatment of Nasolabial Fold Wrinkles.' Journal of the American Academy of Dermatology 62, no. 3 (2009): 448-462.

Neto, Filipe Tenorio Lira, P. V. Bach, R. J. L. Lyra, J. C. Borges Junior, G. T. d. S. Maia, L. C. N. Araujo, and S. V. C. Lima. 'Gods Associated with Male Fertility and Virility.' *Andrology* 7, no. 3 (May 2019): 267–272.

Nikoobakht, Mohammadreza, Alireza Shahnazari, Maedeh Rezaeidanesh, Abdolrasoul Mehrsai, and Gholamreza Pourmand. 'Effect of Penile-Extender Device in Increasing Penile Size in Men with Shortened Penis: Preliminary Results.' *Journal of Sexual Medicine* 8, no. 2 (November 2011): 3188–3192.

NHS, 'Penis Enlargement.' Last modified April 6, 2018. https://www.nhs.uk/live-well/sexual-health/penis-enlargement.

Norman, Greg. 'A man and his dog on a Sunday.' Instagram, November 23, 2020. www.instagram.com/shark_gregnorman.

Oates, Jayson, and Gemma Sharp. 'Nonsurgical Medical Penile Girth Augmentation: Experience-Based Recommendations.' *Aesthetic Surgery Journal* 37, no. 9 (2017): 1032–1038.

Orakwe, J. C., and G. U. Ebuh. '"Oversized" Penile Length in the Black People: Myth or Reality.' *Tropical Journal of Medical Research* 11, no. 1 (2007): 16-18.

Panfilov, Dimitrije E. 'Augmentative Phalloplasty.' *Aesthetic Plastic Surgery* 30, no. 2 (March-April 2006): 183–197.

Pastoor, Hester, and Angela Gregory. 'Penile Size Dissatisfaction.' *The Journal of Sexual Medicine* 17, no. 7 (2020): 1400–1404.

Poulios, Evangelos, Ioannis Mykoniatis, Nikolaos Pyrgidis, Filimon Zilotis, Paraskevi Kapoteli, Dimitrios Kotsiris, Dimitrios Kalyvianakis, and

Dimitrios Hatzichristou. 'Platelet-Rich Plasma (PRP) Improves Erectile Function: A Double-Blind, Randomized, Placebo-Controlled Clinical Trial.' *Journal of Sexual Medicine* 18, no. 5 (May 2021): 926–935.

Prause, Nicole, Jaymie Park, Shannon Leung, and Geoffrey Miller, 'Women's Preferences for Penis Size: A New Research Method Using Selection among 3D Models.' *PLos ONE* 10, no. 9 (2015): 1–17.

Quan, Yuan, Zi-Rui Gao, Xiang Dai, Ling Kuang, Min Zhang, Qing Li, Tao Xu, Xiao-Wei Zhang. 'Complications and Management of Penile Augmentation with Hyaluronic Acid Injection.' *Asian Journal of Andrology* 23 (2021): 392–395.

Radkowsky, Michael. 'Is Size Everything in the Gay Dating/Hooking Scene?' Washington Blade. Last modified January 26, 2018. https://www.washington blade.com/2018/01/26/size-everything-gay-datinghookup-scene.

Rosecker, Ágnes, Noémi Bordás, László Pajor, and Zoltán Bajory. 'Hungarian "Jailhouse Rock": Incidence and Morbidity of Vaseline Self-Injection of the Penis.' *Journal of Sexual Medicine* 10, no. 2 (February 2013): 509–515.

Ryan, Claudine, Tegan Osborne, and Jocelyn Lowinger. 'Using Supplements? You Need to Keep These Things in Mind.' ABC Health and Wellbeing. Last modified May 16, 2016. https://www.abc.net.au/news/health/2016-05-16/supplements-what-you-need-to-know/7408972.

Shaeer, Osama, and Kamal Z. Shaeer. 'The Global Online Sexuality Survey (GOSS): Ejaculatory Function, Penile Anatomy, and Contraceptive Usage among Arabic-Speaking Internet Users in the Middle East.' *Journal of Sexual Medicine* 9, no. 2 (2011): 2152–2163.

Shaeer, Osama, Ditte Skakke, Annamaria Giraldi, Eman Shaeer, and Kamal Shaeer. 'Female Orgasm and Overall Sexual Function and Habits: A Descriptive Study of a Cohort of U.S. Women.' *The Journal of Sexual Medicine* 17, no. 6 (2020): 1–11.

Shar, J., and N. Christopher. 'Can Shoe Size Predict Penile Length?' *BJU International* 90, no. 6 (October 2002): 586–587.

Sickles, Christine, Ali Nassereddin, and Gary P. Gross. *Poly-L-Lactic Acid.* Treasure Island, FL: StatPearls Publishing, 2021. https://www.ncbi.nlm.nih.gov/books/NBK507871.

Siminoski, Kerry, and Jerald Bain. 'The Relationships Among Height, Penile Length, and Foot Size.' *Annals of Sex Research* 6, no. 3 (1993): 231-235.

Stern, Robert. 'Hyaluronan Catabolism: A New Metabolic Pathway.' *European Journal of Cell Biology* 83, no. 7 (2004): 317–325.

Svensøy, Johannes Nordsteien, Valentine Travers, Palle Jörn Sloth Osther. 'Complications of Penile Self-Injections: Investigation of 680 Patients with Complications Following Penile Self-Injections with Mineral Oil.' *World Journal of Urology* 36 (2018): 135–143.

Tae Ahn, Sun, Ji Sung Shim, Woong Jin Bae, Sae Woong Kim, Je Jong Kim, Du Geon Moon. 'Efficacy and Safety of Penile Girth Enhancement Using Hyaluronic Acid Filler and the Clinical Impact on Ejaculation.' *The World Journal of Men's Health* 39 (2021): e23.

Tagata Jinja Official Page. 'Hōnen Matsuri.' Accessed November 24, 2021. http://www.tagatajinja.com/pg28.html.

Thompson, Eliza. 'The 13 Best Superhero Bulges of All Time.' *Cosmopolitan*, April 1, 2014. https://www.cosmopolitan.com/sex-love/g3888/superhero-bulges.

Urology Care Foundation: The Official Foundation of the American Urological Association. 'The Foundation's Recommendation on Penile Augmentation.' Accessed November 1, 2021. https://www.urologyhealth.org/urology-a-z/p/penile-augmentation

Veale, David, Sarah Miles, Sally Bramley, Gordon Muir, and John Hodsoll. 'Am I Normal? A Systematic Review and Construction of Nomograms for Flaccid and Erect Penis Length and Circumference in up to 15,521 Men.' *BJU International* 115, no. 6 (2015): 978–986.

Veale, David, Sarah Miles, Julie Read, Andrea Troglia, Kevan Wylie, and Gordon Muir. 'Sexual Functioning and Behavior of Men with Body Dysmorphic Disorder Concerning Penis Size Compared with Men Anxious about Penis Size and with Controls: A Cohort Study.' *Sexual Medicine* 3, no. 3 (2015): 147–155.

Vicary, Grace Q. 'Visual Art as Social Data: The Renaissance Codpiece.' *Cultural Anthropology* 4, no. 1 (February 1989): 3–25.

Worth, Tammy, 'Does Vagina Size Matter?' WebMD. Last modified July 20, 2011. https://www.webmd.com/women/features/vagina-size.

Wylie, Kevan R., and Ian Eardley. 'Penile Size and the "Small Penis Syndrome".' *BJU International* 99, no. 6 (2007): 1449–1455.

Yang, Dae Yul, Hyun Cheol Jeong, Kyungtae Ko, Seong Ho Lee, Young Goo Lee, and Won Ki Lee. 'Comparison of Clinical Outcomes between Hyaluronic and Polylactic Acid Filler Injections for Penile Augmentation in Men Reporting a Small Penis: A Multicenter, Patient-Blinded/Evaluator-Blinded, Non-Inferiority, Randomized Comparative Trial with 18 Months of Follow-up.' *Journal of Clinical Medicine* 9, no. 4 (April 2020): 1024.

Yuan, J., A.N. Hoang, C.A. Romero, H. Lin, Y. Dai, and R. Wang. 'Vacuum Therapy in Erectile Dysfunction—Science and Clinical Evidence.' *International Journal of Impotence Research* 22 (2010): 211-219.

Zilbergeld, Bernie. *Male Sexuality: A Guide to Sexual Fulfillment*. Boston: Little Brown, 1978.

About the Author

Ingrid Tall is a cosmetic doctor and general practitioner of nearly twenty years, and a life-long lover of day spas from family holidays in Europe with her German mother. As a young doctor, Dr Tall also worked as a medical reporter for Channel 10 News, and in 1993 reported on the new phenomenon of laser resurfacing for facial rejuvenation. This is where her interest in cosmetic medicine began. She has since gone on to create the Aquarius Health and Medical Spa, a luxurious medispa offering the best facials, body scrubs, massages, spa, gym and clinical beauty treatments in Brisbane.

Dr Tall has a continued passion for the evolution of cosmetic medicine and medical journalism, and has been a pioneer in the field of penis filler technology since 2016. She lives with her life partner and their four children in Brisbane, Queensland.

If you would like to know more about penis filler procedures or to find a clinic in your area, please visit:
www.PrivateRenovations.com/FillerOptions

There is a growing demand for this service and we are seeking new professionals to train using our approved programs and become penis enlargement specialists throughout Australia and New Zealand. If you are a doctor, nurse, or similarly medically-trained professional who would like to train in this area, please visit the following link to explore your options:
www.PrivateRenovations.com/Medical

Printed by Libri Plureos GmbH in Hamburg,
Germany